ORTHOTICS: Principles and Practice

Orthotics:
Principles and Practice

G. K. Rose OBE, FRCS

Honorary Consultant Orthopaedic Surgeon,
The Robert Jones and Agnes Hunt Orthopaedic Hospital, Oswestry
and The Royal Shrewsbury Hospitals
Sometime Director of the Orthotic Research
and Locomotor Assessment Unit
and Director of the Gait Assessment Laboratory, Oswestry

WILLIAM HEINEMANN MEDICAL BOOKS
London

Dedication:

To my wife with thanks for her patient understanding

First published in 1986 by William Heinemann Medical Books,
23 Bedford Square, London WC1B 3HH

ISBN 0-433-28280-0

Typeset by Eta Services (Typesetters) Ltd., Beccles, Suffolk
Printed and bound in Great Britain by Anchor Brendon Ltd, Tiptree, Essex

Contents

Acknowledgements

I am very considerably indebted to Miss Katherine Benbow, Occupational Therapist, at the Robert Jones and Agnes Hunt Orthopaedic Hospital, for her comments on upper limb orthoses and her help in preparing some of the figures; to Mr Colin Peacock, MCSP, LBIST for reading and re-reading the text and making useful and practical suggestions; and to Mr J. Stallard, BTech., CEng., MIMech.E, Technical Director of the Orthotic Research and Locomotor Assessment Unit at the Robert Jones and Agnes Hunt Orthopaedic Hospital, who has been a valued colleague for over ten years, contributing importantly to the success of the Unit and who is the author of Appendix A of this volume.

I am also indebted to my secretary, Miss Kirstine Millar, for her patient typing and re-typing of the text.

I am grateful to the Director of the Wallace Collection, London, for permission to publish Fig. 1.1 and to Durr–Fillauer Medical Inc. for permission to publish Fig. 17.8.

For permission to reproduce figures from my contributions to other publications I am grateful to the following:

John Wright & Sons, Bristol for Figs. 2.6, 3.7, 3.8, 3.12, 3.17, 8.7, 8.8, 8.10, 13.4, 13.5, 13.6, 13.9, 13.10, 13.11 and 16.5 from Chapter 32 Orthotics, *Postgraduate Textbook of Clinical Orthopaedics* (Ed. N. H. Harris), 1983.

Her Majesty's Stationery Office, Norwich for Figs. 8.3, 8.9 and 13.12 from *Classification of Orthoses* (DHSS), 1980.

William Heinemann Medical Books Limited, London for Figs. 5.1, 5.2, 5.3, 5.7 and 5.9 from Chapter 52 Principles of splints and orthotics, *Scientific Foundations of Orthopaedics and Traumatology* (Eds R. Owen, J. Goodfellow and P. Bullough), 1980.

Faber and Faber, London for Figs. 2.8, 2.9, 3.19, 13.1, 13.2 and 13.7 from Chapter 7 Foot and knee conditions; Figs. 3.1, 3.2, 3.3, 3.4, 3.9 and 3.14 from Chapter 2 Biomechanics of gait; Figs. 5.12 and 5.13 from Chapter 1 Mechanics of lower limb orthoses (J. Stallard); Fig. 5.15 from Chapter 6 Principles of orthopaedic traction systems (G. K. Rose and E. R. S. Ross), *Cash's Textbook of Orthopaedics and Rheumatology for Physiotherapists* (Ed. P. A. Downie), 1984.

PART I   PRINCIPLES

1

Introduction and definitions

'A skilful surgeon is proficient in his own branch of study, but he does not assume to be equally skilful in mechanical science if he has not made it a subject of study and practice.'

(James Gillingham, Surgical Mechanist, 1888)

This book is an endeavour to identify the scientific bases of orthoses for the better understanding of prescription, measuring and manufacture and to combine these with the accumulated wisdom and expertise of the traditional splint maker/fitter. Clearly, the production of appliances for the treatment of deformities started as empirical, unrecorded acts early in man's history and has been passed from craftsman to pupil on a personalized basis. Consequently, it has long been dominated by consideration of methods of manufacture, often of idiosyncratic devices. Even those called by the same name can differ radically in design, function and efficiency. Written information now tends to come in the form of catalogues of many essentially similar devices, without indication of their mode of action or their relative value. Even recent publications do no more than indicate that a new orthosis or an old one made in different materials is 'good' for this or that medical condition. The present aim is to develop in the reader the ability to recognize the often multiple functions of various forms of orthoses; to appreciate the biological and mechanical principles, so as to be able to recognize and correct orthotic prescription faults; and also to formulate soundly based ideas for developments to meet the challenges of the future.

Recorded examples of splintage appeared in ancient Egyptian and Greek civilizations. By 1564 the product of war, as has often occurred throughout the ages, had a medical by-product: the skill of the armourers in the working and tempering of steel and manufacture of articulations enabled Ambroise Paré, the 'father' of modern surgery, to have made a 'corslet for the correction of a twisted body'. Made of thin steel it was perforated to reduce the weight (he evidently appreciated that such perforations did little to ventilate) and padded to avoid excoriation. He indicated that it should be changed often both in shape and size, particularly for those who are growing to maintain continuous improvement, 'for otherwise instead of doing good one would cause harm'.

Interestingly, armour of the fourteenth century is waisted in a similar manner to the Milwaukee pelvic section; makers had appreciated the problems of taking the considerable weight of the body piece and helmet away from the shoulders and the method of transferring this with optimum comfort to the pelvis (Fig. 1.1).

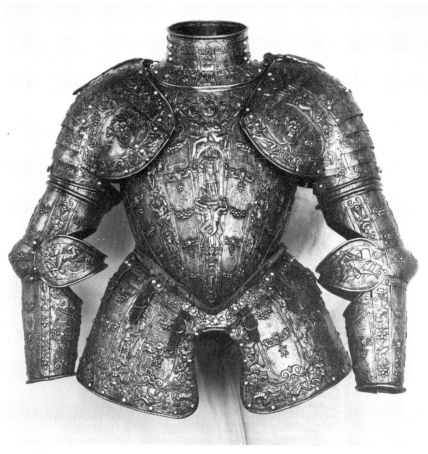

Fig. 1.1 Half armour dated 1519: an example of the 'waisting' found in all armour so that the weight is taken on to the pelvis. Compare this with a Milwaukee and Boston pelvic corset.

In the second half of the eighteenth century, orthopaedic institutions for long-term treatment of patients by exercises and 'instruments' were established in Germany and France. At one of these, plaster-of-Paris casts were taken of distorted limbs prior to treatment in order to demonstrate that change had, in fact, taken place. This was, and is, a valuable discipline which photography has only partially replaced.

From that time on references to appliance makers occurred more frequently, often in catalogues produced by themselves. These often promised assured and near-miraculous cures mixed with philosophical and psychological musings. They were not uncommonly supported by letters of commendation from well-satisfied patients. One has to remember that so little in the way of treatment was available that any device that could restore mobility, often when the doctors had failed, was the greatest possible boon whatever the appearance and to some extent the associated discomfort. In medical literature there were references to the deformities of the famous and infamous and to surgeons with a special interest in this subject. Such a one was Robert Chessher, who died in 1831 and has inscribed on his tombstone:

'permanently distinguished by his liberal benefactions in surgery, anatomy and medicine, he was pre-eminent with an extraordinary skill in mechanism, he made one department of the science peculiarly his own by a new and most successful treatment of spinal deformity and contractions and diseases in the joints and limbs. Machinery was adapted to every different case and patients were attracted from all classes of society and many distant parts of the world. The most perfect cures effected in the most complicated fractures surpassed all former practice and precedent and whilst the tender humanity of his heart and his mild unostentatious manners endeared him to all his numerous acquaintances.'

His technical merit was patently enhanced enormously by his manner of dealing with the patient.

Later, Hugh Owen Thomas, the uncle of Robert Jones and the first of a long line of bone-setters to be medically qualified, not only designed his own splintage but would make and adapt them. His writings on the Thomas bed-knee splint, an early use of continuous traction, contain detailed instructions on the conversion of this to a walking caliper whilst the patient waited and describe instruments used in the process.

In 1839 W. J. Little published an important advance, the use of a surgical procedure to improve the efficiency of splintage. This was percutaneous tenotomy of tendons, which he had learned from Louis Stromeyer of Holland whose patient and apostle he was. It was safe and simple in an age when any surgery was dreaded.

Amongst appliance makers there were obviously very variable levels of skill and understanding, transmitted in an informal apprentice system, often from father to son working as craftsmen who would often prescribe, measure, make and modify the apparatus. They either worked in shops near to major hospitals or, on occasions, hospitals themselves would take on partially handicapped patients to produce appliances in sparsely equipped workshops, often tucked away in some corner or basement where, encouraged by surgeons, they would produce a number of standard and some individualistic appliances. In larger orthopaedic hospitals such workshops were, and generally are, considerably augmented by outside contractors. Patterned on the after-care system introduced by Dame Agnes Hunt at Oswestry in the 1920s, appropriately trained nursing sisters were responsible for the measurement and fitting of patients in after-care clinics scattered throughout a 60-mile radius of the hospital and its workshops. They would then return to the hospital and were generally in daily contact with the manufacturing technicians so that transmission of information was on a highly personal basis despite the distance of the patient from the site of production.

Before the 1914–18 War, orthoses and prostheses were dealt with by the same producers, but the volume of prosthetic demand produced by this war led to the separation of state-financed prosthetic supply from surgical appliances in the UK. With the gradual disappearance of firms supplying mainly private patients, this separation has become almost complete with loss of the valuable cross-fertilization of practices and ideas which exists in most other countries.

In 1948 with the introduction of the National Health Service in the UK further significant changes occurred in the supply of orthoses as in other areas. In consequence:

1.   The Department of Health and Social Services became almost the only

customer. Supply was formalized with independent outside contractors (who at present supply 97 per cent of all orthoses). This is controlled by a complex system of competitive bids and fixed prices, regulations regarding quality of materials and manufacture and administrative arrangements for supply.

2. The statutory obligations of the prescriber, who has to be medically qualified, were defined as to be 'responsible for ensuring that each complete appliance conforms to the prescription and is satisfactory in manufacture, fit and function when fitted to the patient.'

3. A subtle change occurred in the patient–orthotist relationship, the patient acquiring a feeling of a 'right to' an orthosis which satisfied him. This is not always the same as a satisfactory orthosis, and the orthotist must balance patient satisfaction with efficiency.

4. There was a dramatic increase in demand, particularly for surgical belts and footwear.

The definition in (2) is in the main reasonable and emphasizes that the appliance starts with the prescription which requires the same attention and sense of responsibility as that given to prescribing a drug, and ends with the confirmation that the desired end has been achieved. It is, however, unreasonable to expect that, except in very rare cases, a doctor will have had the necessary training in material sciences and design, let alone test facilities, to pass more than a very superficial judgement on manufacture. It is essential that he can transfer this responsibility to a properly trained and qualified orthotist.

This training has been dealt with by the DHSS by the establishment of the Training Council for Orthotists in 1972, replaced by an independent Orthotists and Prosthetists Training and Education Council (OPTEC) in 1981 in England and Wales. In Scotland and Northern Ireland it is controlled by the National Training Centre for Prosthetists and Orthotists. These together provide the now mandatory qualification required by the DHSS if orthotists are to be employed by the contractors to hospitals.

Over the years the number of contractors has diminished sharply and their size has generally increased. The workshops commonly deal with a large number of appliances which can lead both to an improved availability and to use of machinery in addition to more consistent work flow and quality control. It also means that such workshops can be at a considerable distance from the patient supplied. Contact is maintained by orthotists who do not necessarily visit the workshops frequently. The need for accurate gathering of measurement data (including plaster casting) is obviously paramount. It must be in a form readily and accurately understood at the factory. Transmission of this, production of the orthosis and its delivery must be as rapid as possible, all of which requires organization of a high order. In addition, the orthotist must, in the hospital where he works, have a fitting room and small workshop reserved for his use where fitting and modifications can be carried out in conditions that facilitate the work and are reasonable to the patient.

DEFINITIONS

Despite the now universal acceptance internationally of the term 'orthosis' in place of the time-honoured splint, brace or surgical appliance, its origin is obscure. Prosthesis is a much older word (*Shorter Oxford Dictionary*, 1706) and of respectable Greek origin meaning 'in addition'. A prosthesis is, therefore, a replacement or substitute for a missing part. Orthosis is probably a portmanteau word combining orthopaedics and prosthesis. Definition of the term is more difficult. Definition may mean, 'To determine the boundary or limits of, or, alternatively a precise statement of the essential nature of a thing.' The DHSS, using the first approach, defines an orthosis as:

'A device applied direct and externally to the patient's body with the object of supporting, correcting or compensating for an anatomical deformity or weakness, however caused. It may be applied with the additional object of assisting, allowing or restricting movement of the body.'

The essential nature of an orthosis is better defined functionally as:

'An external device designed to apply or remove forces to or from the body in a controlled manner to perform one or both basic functions of:
(a)   control of body motion;
(b)   an alteration or prevention of alteration in the shape of body tissues.'

In order to be complete there must be added to both definitions the warmth and placebo effect.

Control of body motion is used in a strictly mechanical sense and implies:

1.   Absence of motion, i.e. rest in a chosen position.
2.   Limitation of normal range of movement to a chosen degree.
3.   Limitation or avoidance of abnormal movement whilst possibly keeping some or all normal movement.

An orthotist is defined as one qualified by certification to measure for, and to fit all orthoses. Whilst trained to understand manufacturing processes and the implications of these in regard to the prescription and the modification of orthoses, an orthotist is not trained in the manufacturing processes.

An appliance officer has no part in either function of an orthotist and is solely concerned with the administrative aspects of supply and payments for orthoses. Some appliance officers do fulfil a dual role, usually to a limited degree, e.g. fitting of belts, but only by virtue of special training and certification.

The term orthotics covers the theory and practice of prescription, fitting, design, assessment and production of orthoses. The ideal supply situation requires three main components:

1.   An interested medical prescriber who has a clear idea of the aim of treatment, orthotic potentials and limitations, who is willing in appropriate circumstances to make decisions based on full ongoing discussions with the orthotist and other sources of relevant information including patients and/or parents, physiotherapists and occupational therapists, and who will assess the value of the results on a wide basis including independence and cosmesis.
2.   An orthotist with an up-to-date knowledge of the science and art of orthotics. Science includes the properties and limitations of materials, a confident grasp of static mechanics and an insight into dynamics to be able to appreciate the mechanical stresses produced in the orthosis, at the

interface and within the patient. He or she must have a basic understanding of the medical conditions to be treated, and be able to identify the orthotic implications. The art is patient management and includes the ethics and psychology of the patient relationship, an explanation of the orthotic function, support during the inevitable initial (and sometimes permanent) limitations which all orthoses impose in addition to their benefits, and the ability to minimize these by a variety of small measures.

3.   A manufacturer willing and able constantly to upgrade methods of production and quality control to provide a fast assured service to the patient requiring a minimum modification.

The patient is the centre of the whole organization but must also make a positive contribution by accepting the inevitable 'running in' period. They will do so most easily if the period is short and if all professional contributors demonstrate their competence and efficiency.

2

Mechanical principles, biological response and biological context

MECHANICAL PRINCIPLES

There now exist so many sources of detailed basic information on mechanical principles orientated to medical needs that it is not proposed to reiterate them comprehensively (Cochran, 1982; Frankel and Burstein, 1970; Frost, 1973; Williams and Lissner, 1977).

Easy, confident familiarity with statics is essential and immediately rewarding. It is by no means a difficult subject. Dynamics is more difficult, but even if calculations are to remain in the province of design orthotists and bioengineers, knowledge of the implications of the very substantial rise in force due to movement and inertia must be well appreciated. It is important that all working in this field must have a precise common language where words like 'stabilization' have one meaning only. At present to the orthopaedic surgeon this means a process of surgical stiffening whilst to the engineer it has an entirely different meaning. Whilst it is an inescapable fact that Newton's laws of motion apply to every body animate and inanimate at all times, there has been a strange reluctance by doctors whose training and practice is orientated to biological concepts, to take this into account in considering the treatment of the human body. Of course, it has a capacity for adaptation and self-repair not present in machines; but the demands on these biological processes can be reduced by the use of Newton's laws, particularly the third, with great advantage both in healing and in design of orthoses. Key words are force and energy.

Force is a vector and has, therefore, both direction and magnitude. Multiple forces can be represented graphically, and manipulated to demonstrate the resultant force or moment. Applied at a right angle to a fixed surface, a compressive mechanical stress called pressure is generated, the degree of which can be quantified. Acting in the line of the surface, shear stress is produced which is much more difficult to measure. Both pressure and shear are of particular importance in regard to the skin interface and subcutaneous tissue.

In any practical situation several forces will be at work and the ultimate effect of these can be determined by resolution, either into single force or a turning moment. Where the sum of these forces and/or moments is nil the system is said to be in equilibrium. Stability is a limited element of equilibrium applied both to solid bodies and to segmented structures. Although subdivided into unstable, stable, neutral and metastable (Fig. 2.1), it is stable stability which is of first importance in orthotics. It is most easily understood in a solid body (Fig. 2.2) which if displaced slightly will automatically return to its resting state. If the centre of gravity (more accurately designated the centre of mass) passes outside the support area it becomes unstable and support would be needed to prevent the object falling over. The degree of support and therefore the pressure applied to the body mounts rapidly as the angle increases.

In a multi-segmented body, it is the centre of mass of all segments above the axis under consideration which has to be considered. For example, a patient with weak extensors of the hips has to place the resultant centre of mass of head, trunk and arms behind the hip joint to avoid falling forwards (Fig. 2.3). It can be appreciated, therefore, that a deformity that is mobile and can be brought back to an inherently stable position, as in the slightly hyperextended knee, can be retained in that position by the application of, theoreti-

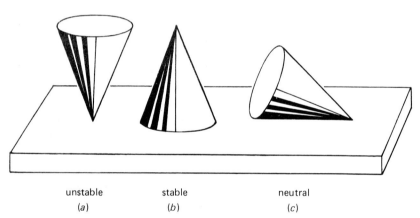

| unstable | stable | neutral |
| (a) | (b) | (c) |

Fig. 2.1 Forms of stability. (a) Unstable: theoretically this position can be held but the slightest extraneous force will displace it. (b) Stable: provided that the centre of mass remains within the support area, it can be tilted but will return to the resting position. (c) Neutral: if moved the object will remain in the new position.

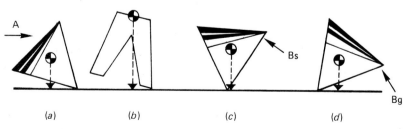

| (a) | (b) | (c) | (d) |

Fig. 2.2 Centre of mass in relationship to support area. (a) When force A is removed, cone returns to stable position. (b) The gait situation identical to (a). (c) Unstable position requiring small supporting force Bs. (d) As (c) but supportive force is now great (Bg).

cally, no force. When allowance is made for slight disturbances of equilibrium due to movement this stable position can be maintained with a minimum force. There are consequently no interface pressure problems. In contrast, where a deformity is only partially correctable, the situation is one of support, not stabilization, and interface problems can become difficult to manage. The orthosis may be unacceptably painful in the patient with sensation and unsafe in one without.

In assessing the effect of these forces, the greatest problem is to make sure that *all* are considered. An aid to doing this is the free body diagram. Any complex system, as for example that below the knee when a below-knee orthosis is worn, can be resolved by considering each component separately in a variety of chosen positions of function. Three are shown in Fig. 2.4 but the exercise could also be repeated in the coronal as well as the sagittal plane. The salient points in this case are considered in some detail under below-knee orthoses, but some important considerations are:

1. The length of moment arms in relationship to interface pressure.
2. The change in direction of the force applied to the upper area during stance.
3. The deforming forces applied to the orthosis after heel rise.

Such diagrams immediately give a better understanding of the changes that occur during gait, inherent limitations, and indications of problem-solving needs.

A full understanding of this technique is essential for the designer or modifier of orthoses. The prescriber only needs an understanding of the principles and results. The free body diagram does re-emphasize that all three components of the mechanical system which operates when an orthosis is used need consideration in respect of the results of the forces, intermittent and constant, within each, i.e. those:

1. Within the orthosis which can distort or break it.
2. At the essential interface between orthosis, skin and subcutaneous tissue which form a combined pressure/shear-resisting layer.
3. Within the treated part. It is important that if a force is being used to modify body shape it is applied only to the area of deformity. Furthermore, if this area is resistant to force it will then react at other less robust points. A notable example is the deformation of the jaw in the older type of Milwaukee splint when passive traction was exerted between jaw and pelvis. Growing tissues are particularly vulnerable in this respect.

A force commonly neglected in these considerations is that generated by muscular activity. This can be used beneficially, particularly if an appropriate orthosis can be provided for it to react against. The modern Milwaukee orthosis is an example of this (see pages 51 and 94) as is the appropriate plaster facilitating mobilization of finger joints (Fig. 2.5).

It is also in the difficult area of modification of body shape that thinking in terms of energy is most valuable. Work is force times distance moved; energy is the capacity to do work and exists in many forms: thermal, atomic, electromagnetic, chemical and mechanical. Mechanical energy may be of the following kinds:

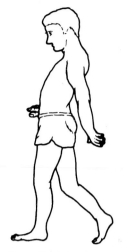

Fig. 2.3 Typical posture assumed by a patient suffering from muscular dystrophy. The centre of mass of the head, trunk and arms is kept behind the hip joint during the whole gait cycle to avoid falling forwards because of profound weakness of hip extensor muscles.

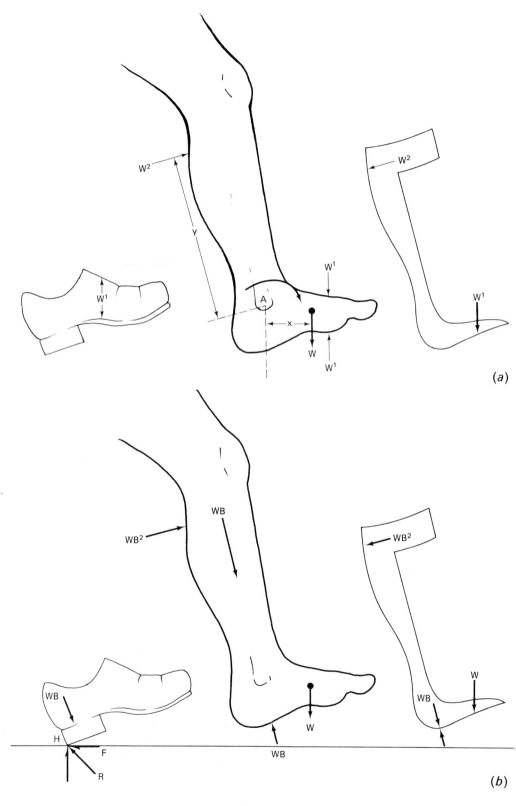

(a)

(b)

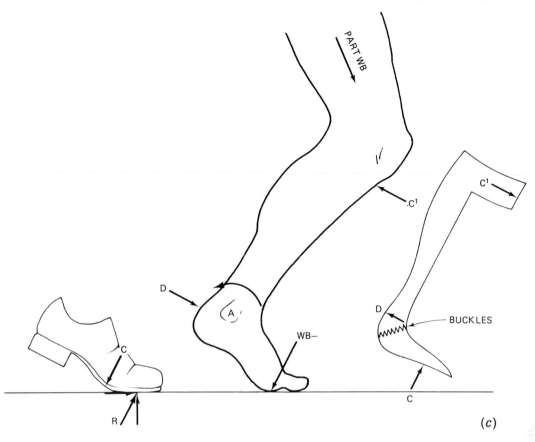

Fig. 2.4 The three components in the use of a plastic below knee orthosis used for foot drop (AFO, plantar resist). The shoe, leg and orthosis are considered separately at three chosen points in the gait cycle: (a) during swing phase, (b) at heel strike, and (c) at end-of-stance phase. W is weight of foot, which during swing has a moment about the ankle and reacts against the orthosis at W^1. This would push the orthosis down the leg but when the shoe is on, the orthosis in turn presses on the sole and this force, W^1, is transmitted to the upper over the dorsum of the foot. In these circumstances $W \times X$ equals the moment about the ankle axis A and the equilibrium is maintained by the moment $W^2 \times Y$. The longer Y is, the smaller W^2 will be. In any case, because the weight of the foot is small the length Y is at this time not significant but the situation changes radically once the stance phase begins. WB approximates to the body weight, it keeps the orthosis in place relative to the foot and the shoe is not required. The heel of the shoe contacts the ground and is prevented from slipping forwards by friction F. This produces the final resultant R which can be measured on a force plate. Whilst the weight of the foot still produces a moment as before around the ankle, to this is added the much larger moment about the point of heel contact H and together these are resisted by a force perpendicular to the top of the calf, WB^2. In these circumstances it is imperative that the distance Y should be as long as possible to avoid both interface pressure and wasting of the underlying muscles with prolonged use.

At the end of the stance phase there is a further change. A proportion of WB presses now against the anterior orthotic cuff, C^1, and if this is not padded there will be discomfort here as the force is high. It presses the front edge of the orthosis against the inside of the shoe sole which reacts with the ground. This in turn causes a moment around the heel angle of the orthosis and buckling because the axis of this does not usually correspond with that of the ankle. Clearly this can be a source of considerable discomfort and requires consideration from the point of view of design.

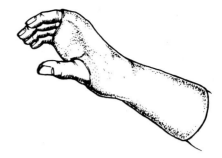

Fig. 2.5 Extended Colles' type plaster cast for mobilizing stiff proximal interphalangeal joints. This concentrates flexor muscle activity on the affected joints only.

1. Potential energy which exists by virtue of position relative to a datum line, e.g. someone standing up stores potential energy in relationship to the floor and this will be returned if they sit down, a fact well appreciated by all who have done this in an uncontrolled manner!
2. Kinetic energy by virtue of movement which increases with the speed of movement, a fact known to anyone who has received a blow from a cricket ball.
3. Inertial energy which is that used to overcome the property of a body to resist change of motion; either to stop a moving body or to move one at rest requires greater energy than that needed to keep it in steady motion. This is also time-related so the faster the stopping or starting is done, the greater the energy required.
4. Strain or stored energy; the absorption or release of energy by virtue of change of shape. When a corrective device is applied by a patient it will be efficient only if the application requires the injection of some energy from the patient's arm muscles which will then be released in stretching the affected tissues. It means that there must be some element of discomfort at the interface and that once this stretching has occurred the orthosis will have no further function until it has been readjusted, by modification of the shape of a passive device or adjustment of springs or elastic in an active one.

BIOLOGICAL RESPONSE

The biological response to orthotic treatment is fundamental to the study of this subject, particularly in relation to skin and the effects of heat.

Skin

Pressure, which is force per unit area, can be reduced either by increasing the area of application or diminishing the force. Excessive pressure will damage:

1. The epidermis and dermis.
2. The superficial circulation.

Intermittent pressure will first provoke a benign thickening and formation of callosities if applied slowly. This is a protective reaction and if backed by a normal subcutaneous tissue gives no symptoms. Some forms of relatively rigid plastic insoles supplied for the treatment of flat feet for children can give rise to this and if the child has no complaint the parent can be reassured. Even quite thickened areas will completely disappear when the cause is removed. If applied quickly and vigorously over a short period the familiar blister will appear. Some areas have evolved naturally for sustaining pressure and these should be the area of choice, if possible, for the application of interface forces. Areas to be avoided are those where, either naturally or due to pathology, a sharp bony prominence is covered by a thin or traumatized subcutaneous tissue. Shear stress is particularly troublesome in such areas. Normally the fibro-fatty subcutaneous layer allows the skin to slide over underlying bony points (and is especially modified in the foot and hand to be extremely efficient in this) and thereby absorb this potentially destructive force. This mechanism is particularly well illustrated in the foot where the situation is analogous to the track of a military tank. The skin, like the track, remains stationary relative to the contact area whilst the bone rolls forwards within it (Fig. 2.6). Adherence of the skin to bone or thinned fibrous tissue reduces the ability to make this excursion and subcutaneous tearing will occur so that the situation progressively deteriorates. In neuropathic ulceration this will prevent healing despite the optimization of pressure. The solution is to transfer the shear from this area to the shoe–floor interface by the provision of a correctly designed rigid rocker sole.

Continuous pressure will damage the superficial circulation particularly

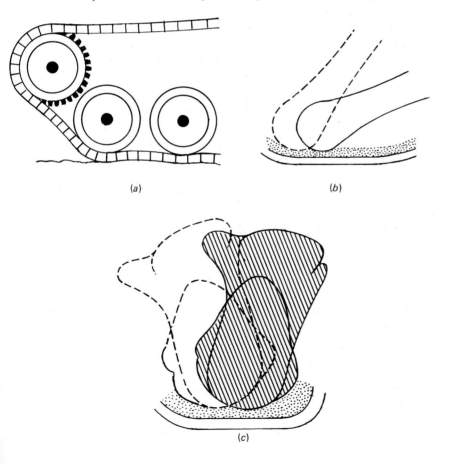

(a)

(b)

(c)

Fig. 2.6 (a) A military tank track. The wheels rotate but the track is still relative to the ground. (b) An analogous situation in the sagittal plane of the metatarsal head, (c) The os calcis in the coronal plane.

where the function of this is reduced by diabetes, rheumatoid arthritis and other diseases that affect the vascularity of a limb. The secondary effects include ulceration or local gangrene. Intermittent pressure is tolerated at much higher levels.

The effects of heat

General

Large orthoses, particularly of plastic, which closely conform to the body can reduce the percentage of the body area available for cooling. This is particularly important in hot climates. Heat exhaustion may occur, although this is only a real possibility where a very large area is covered as in some of the combined body–legs orthoses for spina bifida.

Local effects

Heat retention (calefaction)
Discomfort from heat retention—as in the use of thermoplastic materials in vacuum-formed footwear for rheumatoid arthritis—is a relatively common cause for complaint or even rejection. In patients with a reduced peripheral circulation a temperature rise can increase the oxygen need of the tissues at a proportionately greater rate than the increased circulation can deliver. The situation can then become dangerous and precipitate local necrosis. On the other hand, warmth has been claimed as an important beneficial effect of orthoses, particularly in older people.

Sweating and maceration
Sweating and maceration of the skin increases the vulnerability to trauma and hence the invasion of microorganisms, including bacteria, yeasts and fungi which normally inhabit the skin. It is not always realized that in footwear only 1 per cent of the sweat normally produced in a day transpires through the sole if this is leather. Plastic soling material, therefore, makes little difference to the situation. The remaining 99 per cent is only partly removed, some through the material of the upper; leather is most efficient in this respect. The major loss occurs by the movement of the foot within the shoe causing a pumping effect, and some through the wick effect of the sock. Cotton is vastly superior to man-made fibres for this. At the end of the day with all these systems working together a proportion of sweat still remains in the shoe; this is not dried out completely during the night. This can easily be established by accurate weighing of the shoe and implies that for foot and footwear health, particularly where the patient has a pathological vulnerability, the same pair of shoes should not be worn on successive days.

THE BIOLOGICAL CONTEXT OF ORTHOTIC TREATMENT

In considering the need for orthotic prescription and in assessing the results of treatment, variations in physique and age are commonly ignored.

Variations in physique

These are part of an individual's genetic makeup and although encompassing wide variations in shape cannot be regarded as abnormal and cannot generally be changed by orthotic treatment. Physique is also ethnically related. The problem has been to judge at what point wide variations from the average pass into a pathological condition. Judgements are often made on the basis of a condition not looking 'right' and such judgements are often based on individual observer prejudice. Harris (Harris and Beath, 1947) recounts in his excellent survey of the feet of 3500 soldiers, carefully measured and documented and then followed up for functional ability, that in one area of Canada 'flat foot' was nine times as prevalent as elsewhere. However, the objective survey showed that these 'flat foot' sufferers were a typical sample as compared with the others.

As a base line for understanding of this problem, Sheldon (Sheldon *et al.*, 1940; Sheldon, 1954) subdivided the general population into three main groups which he called somatotypes (Fig. 2.7). Whilst these blend into each other the representative characteristics of each group were:

1. *Ectomorphs*—Ectomorphs are relatively tall with a thin narrow chest and abdomen, relatively little muscle and subcutaneous fat and large skin area. They tend to have hypermobile joints with orthotic implications. Like all groups their internal organs, the heart for example, have similar characteristics.
2. *Mesomorphs*—Mesomorphs have broad shoulders and chest, heavily muscled arms and legs with the distal segments (forearms and calves) strong in relationship to the proximal (upper arms and thighs). They are not necessarily fat (overweight is independent of the somatotype) and characteristically have little subcutaneous fat with a small anteroposterior dimension.
3. *Endomorphs*—Endomorphs are as near spherical as is humanly possible. They have considerable subcutaneous fat but this does not simply make them obese subjects, for their front-to-back diameter of thorax and pelvis is greater than the side-to-side diameter. This suggests that they have a higher proportion of fat cells in their body than the average whilst mesomorphs have a lower ratio of fat cells.

Tanner (1964) in his somatotyping of Olympic athletes demonstrated, using a sophisticated classification based on this system, that those taking part in any one particular event had similar typing. Half of those found in a general population study were not represented at all and these were distributed between extreme ectomorphy through to endomorphy. In illness (particularly neurological) and in injury, one can expect significant variation in response to treatment whether orthotic or physical therapy depending on type.

Mechanically, as sometimes seen architecturally, strange-looking structures may have no abnormal internal or external stresses. For example, the fact that a pathological flat foot has a marked 'valgus' with the internal malleolus

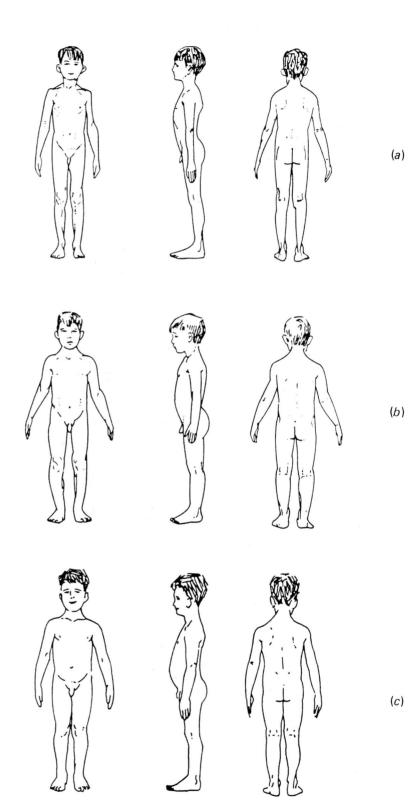

Fig. 2.7 Sheldon's somatotypes:
(a) ectomorphs, (b) mesomorphs,
(c) endomorphs.

extremely prominent does not mean that all feet with a similar valgus are pathological and functional assessment may reveal no abnormality.

Variations with age

The child's skeleton is not simply a scaled-down version of the adult (Fig. 2.8) and inevitably differential growth occurs. For example, there is a natural history of change in foot posture (Fig. 2.9), of genu valgum (Fig. 2.10) and genu

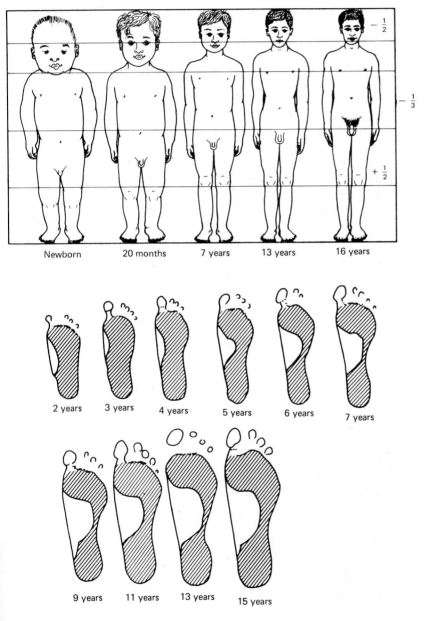

Newborn   20 months   7 years   13 years   16 years

Fig. 2.8 Change in body proportions with age.

2 years   3 years   4 years   5 years   6 years   7 years

9 years   11 years   13 years   15 years

Fig. 2.9 Natural history of change in foot posture.

varum (Fig. 2.11). It is well recognized that in the infantile form of scoliosis almost all recover without treatment. An orthosis used in these situations can acquire an unwarranted reputation for efficiency.

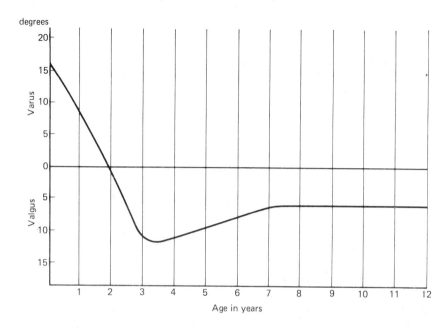

Fig. 2.10 Natural change from genu varum to valgum with ageing.

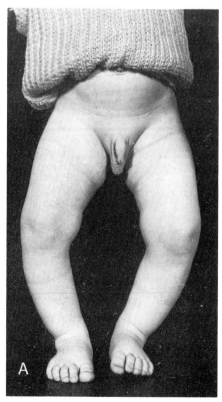
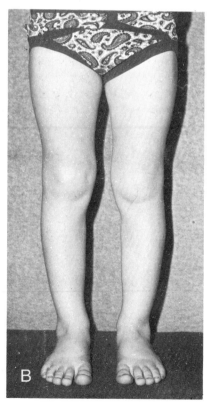

Fig. 2.11 The considerable change that can occur in a patient with genu valgum, untreated for 3 years.

3

The essential components of gait

TERMINOLOGY

Walking is divided into two obvious phases—swing and stance—occurring simultaneously in opposite legs and sequentially in the same leg. There are two phases of double stance, each about 13 per cent of the total cycle and starting at the commencement of toe and the heel rocker of each leg. Walking becomes running when there are no double-stance phases. Arbitrary division of each phase is made as shown in Fig. 3.1.

Stride length is the ground covered between the beginning and end of one completed phase of one leg, i.e. start of swing through stance to the beginning of swing. To move in a straight line this must be equal on both sides. Step length is the distance one foot moves in front of the other and step lengths can be unequal or even negative.

Without an understanding of the fundamental features of gait, no satisfactory understanding of lower-limb orthoses is possible and this is particularly the case in the design of new orthoses. Gait is a highly complex activity and it is only possible to indicate those factors directly related to orthoses. The mandatory components for any form of locomotion whether animate or inanimate are:

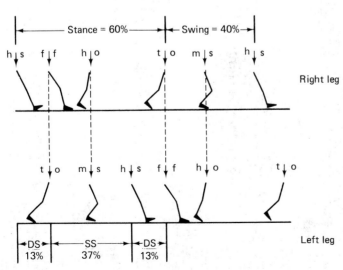

Fig. 3.1 Proportions of gait cycle. Note the relationships of one leg with the other and that twice in each phase of walking double stance (DS) occurs when both touch the ground and share the load in varying degrees. SS = single stance; hs = heel strike; ff = foot flat; ho = heel off; to = toe off; ms = mid swing.

1. Stabilization of a multi-segmented structure—the skeleton, both intrinsically and extrinsically.
2. Propulsion by provision of an internal primary source of energy, namely muscle. This energy is then manipulated in the most efficient way to produce an external reaction.
3. A complex control system to maintain (1) and (2).

STABILIZATION

Intrinsic stabilization

This is the prevention of collapse of the multi-segmented skeleton. When standing this is normally achieved, not as was once thought by postural muscle tone (through continuous asynchronous activity of muscle fibres) but basically by balancing one bone on another. This may be demonstrated despite the shape of the skeleton, even with spinal curves (Fig. 3.2). Obviously such stability is precarious and has to be maintained by appropriate controlled injection of muscle activity. This system results in a high level of energy conservation compared with continuous muscular effort (Fig. 3.3). In the absence of pain it is minimization of energy expenditure that dictates the mode of

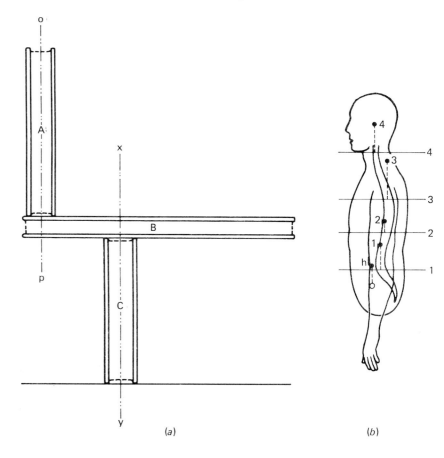

Fig. 3.2 (a) Three books in a balanced, stable position. General centre of mass (gravity) line x–y is irrelevant when considering the stability of the 'joint' between books A and B. The centre of mass of A lies in line o–p, it is within the support area of A which is therefore stable on B. (b) Applying this to the human form, it is clear that the only relevant centre of mass in relationship to any particular joint is that of the portion of the body above that joint. Lines 2, 3 and 4 show thoraco-lumbar, mid-thoracic and mid-cervical articulations, respectively, and it will be seen that the relevant centres of mass are situated above their respective joints. Although the human spine is curved, each segment is in fact balanced on the one below it and requires no muscular effort to support this. h = hip.

(a)   (b)

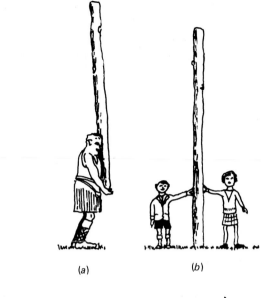

Fig. 3.3 Energy saving of muscle used to balance as opposed to support. The energy required to hold the caber in (a) is clearly much greater than in (b). Should the caber tend to tilt, however, it requires a high level of controlled feedback from the children and with this the caber can be restored to stability with very slight energy expenditure.

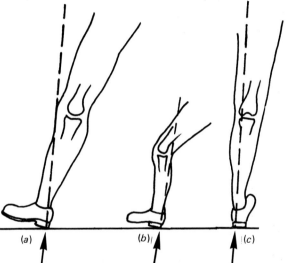

Fig. 3.4 Vector of ground reaction in two planes. (a) Note that in this particular case it passes in front of the knee joint and causes an extending moment which will stabilize the joint without muscle action. (b) If the knee was flexed due to a contracture, the moment will be flexing. (c) In the transverse plane the vector passes through the medial compartment of the knee, which is normal.

walking and it is important to appreciate that this may result in a limp. This limp can be abolished by orthotic modification, but if this increases the energy cost it may then be unacceptable to the patient.

In standing, the force applied to the system is that of gravity working at right angles to the floor. In walking the forces, a combination of gravity and those generated by movement, provide a ground reaction (vector) which is oblique for much of the gait cycle (Fig. 3.4) and it is the relationship of the ground reaction to various joints which determines their inherent stability at any time. For example, given a normal range of knee movement allowing a slight hyperextension it is possible to maintain knee stability in walking with a paralysed quadriceps muscle on level ground by keeping the vector ahead of the knee axis. On sloping ground, particularly away from the patient, the rela-

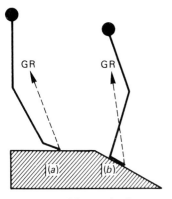

Fig. 3.5 (a) Stability on a level surface is more assured when there is an equinus at the ankle which places the ground reaction (GR) forward. It has the disadvantage of relatively lengthening the leg and therefore increasing the energy requirement for the 'uphill' phase of stance. (b) When going down a slope the GR becomes a flexor moment, and an orthosis is necessary to achieve stability.

tionship of the force vector to the knee is changed adversely (Fig. 3.5). If knee joints have a flexion contracture for any reason in an unparalysed patient, stability has to be maintained either by increased muscular activity with consequent rise in energy expenditure or by an orthosis. The earliest and perhaps the commonest use of orthoses in the lower limb is to provide intrinsic stability. In high lesions affecting all joints, orthoses may be single or combined—the total exoskeleton (Fig. 3.6) or a combination of knee-stabilizing orthoses with the use of crutches to stabilize the hip (Fig. 3.7).

Extrinsic stability

Extrinsic stability is the prevention of falling of the intrinsically stabilized skeleton. This requires that the centre of mass of the whole body remains within the support area which may be increased in a swivel walker by providing enlarged footplates (Fig. 3.8) or by the other effect of crutches (Fig. 3.7). In the normal dynamic situation of walking static extrinsic stabilization is not achieved (Fig. 3.9). The centre of gravity would need to be moved over each foot in turn to achieve this resulting in an excessive movement of it both laterally and upwards. It is, in fact, moved towards the support foot storing potential energy which is returned as it then falls back (Fig. 3.10). During the brief time interval whilst this occurs (normally about 400 ms) the swing leg is moved forward. If the adduction of the hip cannot be controlled during this process the centre of mass may tend to pass outside the support foot. The sys-

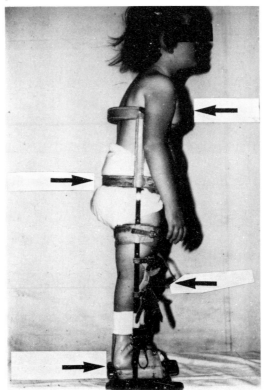

Fig. 3.6 Exoskeleton of the swivel walker type. Four forces are required, as shown, to provide intrinsic stabilization of ankles, knees and hips. It will be appreciated that these are two sets of overlapping three-point fixations.

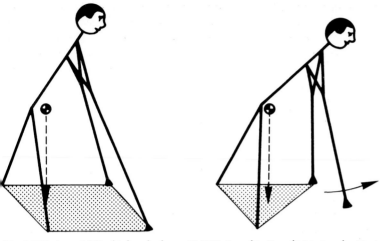

Fig. 3.7 The knee stabilized in long leg braces (KAFO). A combination of intrinsic and extrinsic stability is provided. The crutches prevent the hips from flexing forward whilst the support area (shaded) remains large even when one crutch is being moved forwards.

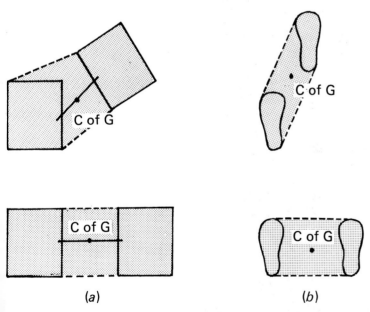

Fig. 3.8 Large footplates upon a swivel walker used to increase extrinsic stabilization (a) compared with the normal support area (b). Note that (a) is very stable in all phases of gait, whereas in (b) with the stride the centre of gravity (mass) comes nearer to the edge and requires, therefore, more refined feedback and control.

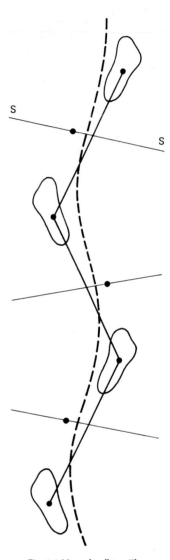

Fig. 3.9 Normal walking. The dotted line is the path of the centre of mass (gravity). Note that it does not go over each foot as this assumes support. S–S is the shoulder line and moves in the opposite direction to the pelvis.

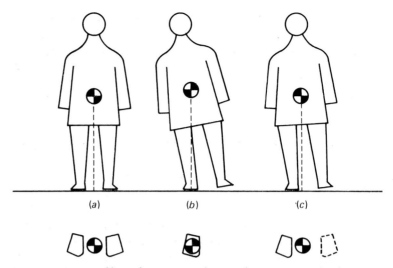

Fig. 3.10 (a) A static stable standing position with centre of mass (gravity) within the support area of the two feet. (b) Static stable position with single-foot support area. Clearly not as assured as (a). (c) Dynamic stable position, not in itself stable but will fall back to stable position (a).

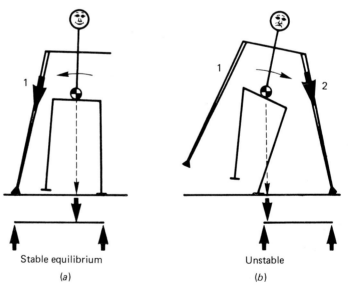

Fig. 3.11 Diagrammatic representation of (a) stable type of equilibrium achieved with a rigid hip guidance orthosis. An injection of energy down crutch 1 is required to lift the foot from the ground and this energy is then largely returned as the system, under the influence of gravity, returns to the two-foot stance. (b) When the orthosis is flexible the centre of mass (gravity) passes beyond the support leg, the second injection of energy is then required through crutch 2 in order to prevent the patient falling or producing an unsafe broken-rhythm form of gait.

tem is then unstable, and if no force is injected the patient will fall sideways. The best control is preventative—for example, in the complete paraplegic the provision of an appropriately rigid orthosis crossing the hip, as in a hip guidance orthosis (see page 186). If it occurs an additional injection of energy can be made by a crutch on the same side (Fig. 3.11(a)) but the total energy cost is then increased and the rhythm of forward progression adversely affected.

INTERNALLY PRODUCED ENERGY AND EXTERNAL REACTION

Although some contribution of muscular energy from some source in the body must be made in any form of gait, bipedal or quadripedal, it is the optimal transference of this energy through the system at appropriate times through its various forms that will determine the efficiency of gait; and this applies to the handicapped assisted by an orthosis. A few exhausting dragging steps cannot be defined as walking and will be rejected by the patient as soon as he or she has a free choice. If one examines a simple example this transfer of energy between different forms becomes clear.

In a straight leg gait primary muscular energy is injected during the 'uphill' phase to produce a potential energy balance (Fig. 3.12) which is then returned

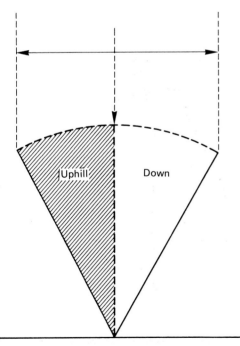

Fig. 3.12 Diagram of stance movement of a leg held in a long leg brace (KAFO). During the uphill phase the centre of mass (gravity) of the body is raised and muscular energy must be provided. It is transformed into potential energy at the peak and released as kinetic energy in the downhill phase and during this period requires no further muscular activity.

without further muscular effort during the 'downhill' phase. During this descent the potential energy is transferred into kinetic and this in turn into inertial which will advantageously spill over to assist the 'uphill phase' of the other leg. The potential energy here is related to the weight of the body. In the swing phase it is related to the weight of the leg (Fig. 3.13).

By placing the hips forward of the foot when this is then raised from the ground it will swing forward to the vertical as its potential energy becomes kinetic and onwards to be landed ahead of the hip. No muscular energy is required to be produced in the leg to achieve this. Just prior to grounding, this leg comes to a standstill in space and this releases inertial energy which assists forward movement of the body. It should be noted that at this point that there is no 'push off'.

In normal gait this energy transfer or flux is reflected in the comparatively little muscular activity which occurs in the legs (Fig. 3.14). That which occurs is of two types—concentric and eccentric. Only concentric, contraction with shortening, is concerned with forward movement whilst eccentric, tightening occurring with lengthening, fulfils the important role of shock absorption. A brief, transient intermediate stage, when no change in length occurs, can bridge the two main activities. This is known as an isometric stage.

It may seem very obvious that all this activity will fail to move the body forward if the resultant force at the contact area cannot react against the ground, but in design of orthoses for the paraplegic definitive steps may need

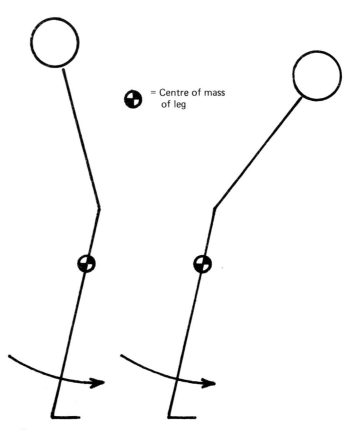

Fig. 3.13 Use of centre of mass (gravity) of leg to produce muscle-free swing. The essential feature is that the hip is ahead of the foot and not that the hip is either extended or flexed.

= Centre of mass
of leg

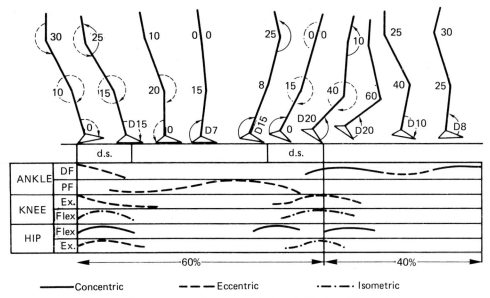

Fig. 3.14 Joint movements and muscle activity during gait cycle. d.s. = double stance; PF = plantar flexion, DF = dorsiflexion, Ex. = extension; Flex = flexion.

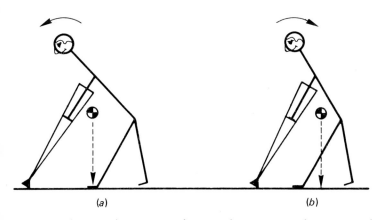

Fig. 3.15 (a) The centre of mass (gravity) of system within support area. The patient is tending to fall forwards and the reaction of the crutches against the ground enables the muscular energy of the arms and trunk to be applied in order to raise the centre of gravity of the body during the uphill phase. In (b) the centre of mass (gravity) is behind the support area and there will be a posterior fall-out unless the swing leg is grounded in the position it has just left. Use of the crutches and arm muscles are powerless to prevent this as there is no ground reaction.

to be taken in order to achieve this. As will be seen in Fig. 3.15 unless the hip flexion in a hip guidance orthosis is limited, the centre of gravity will fall behind the stance leg, the crutches which are relied on to transmit the muscle energy of the arms to the ground will move away from it and forward movement becomes impossible.

CONTROL MECHANISM

In order for stability and propulsion to be maintained, very considerable levels of servo-control mechanism are necessary to maintain the pattern of energy production and flux through various forms and body components. Where controls are deficient naturally they may be produced orthotically, for example, in the articulation used to programme joint movements (hip guidance articulations) or even in the production of a rhythmic noise as an external feedback (with swivel walkers).

COMPONENTS OF GAIT

Maximum efficiency in usage of energy during ambulation is achieved by reducing the necessary movement of the body centre of mass in all planes for functional progression to a minimum. Optimum amplitude, in any given situation, is determined by the use of movements conveniently designated 'components of gait', which unlike 'components of locomotion' are not all mandatory but can be used in various combinations. They are:

1. Flexion–extension action of the swing leg—a pendulum.
2. Vaulting action of the stance leg.
3. At the pelvis in three planes, i.e. horizontal rotation, lateral movement and

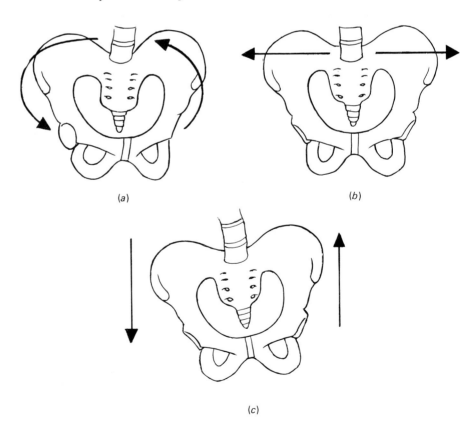

(a)

(b)

(c)

Fig. 3.16 Variations in pelvic components of gait. (a) Horizontal rotation. (b) Lateral translation. (c) Vertical rotation.

vertical rotation in the coronal plane to produce rise and fall of each hip in turn (Fig. 3.16). This is much concerned with the bipedal alternation of stance and swing gait. The ability to get one foot off the ground and to swing this saves the high friction energy cost of the 'drag-to' type of pathological gait. In the design of orthoses for paraplegia consideration has to be given to the optimum way to achieve this as indicated later under hip guidance orthosis and swivel walkers.

4. At the knee, where two phases of flexion occur during the gait cycle: the first on heel contact concerned in the main with shock absorption, and the second prior to toe-off and during swing gait concerned with the clearance of the swing leg. During stance the knee movement has a profound effect on regulating the rise and fall of the centre of mass. Complete loss of movement here causes a rise in energy consumption of some 25 per cent (Fishman *et al.*, 1982).

5. At the foot–ankle complex there are three 'rockers' (Fig. 3.17), although occurring successively there is some overlap:

    (a) The heel rocker in barefoot walking is an impact shock-absorbing mechanism because of the calcaneo-contact rolling effect (see page 218) combined with the controlled plantar flexion of the foot to resist the moment about the heel (Fig. 3.18). Foot slap and consequent impact on the forefoot are avoided. In addition it carries forward the shank, and the amount of progression is increased by the heel of the footwear.

    (b) The ankle rocker is the most important element in forward progression and pathological or orthotic limitation of this has important implications for modification of the gait cycle, mostly adverse but occasionally beneficial in that such limitations can be used to enhance knee extension and therefore stability (see Fig. 3.5).

    (c) The toe rocker enables the transition between stance and swing phase to occur smoothly and is very much related to the shear stress relief in the forefoot.

Within the foot there exists the plantar fascia mechanism, which is shortened and tightened each time extension of the phalanges occurs, which normally happens twice in each gait cycle. This is because of its anatomy; it is inserted at one end of the os calcis and anteriorly divided into five slips which are attached to the bases of the proximal phalanges (Fig. 3.19). At heel strike active extension of the toes occurs which causes arch rise most markedly on

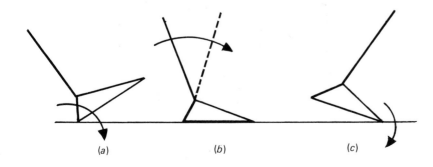

(a)   (b)   (c)

Fig. 3.17 The three rockers: (a) heel, (b) ankle and (c) toe. Note that the shank moves forwards during all rockers and also downwards in (a) and upwards in (c).

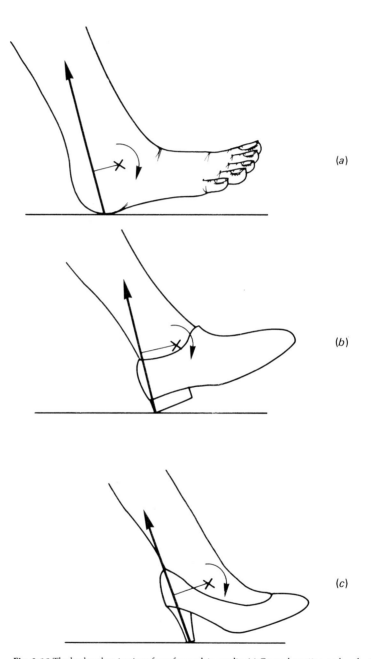

Fig. 3.18 The heel rocker: tracings from force-plate results. (a) Ground reaction on barefoot heel contact producing a plantar flexing moment about the ankle X which is resisted during movement by the eccentric activity of the dorsi-flexor muscles. (b) A man's shoe heel showing increase in moment. (c) This moment will be increased by up to 40 per cent with the highest women's heels. The effect, however, is mitigated by the forward placing of the heel contact relative to the foot. At the same time the movement forward of the ankle in space may be increased up to 100 per cent.

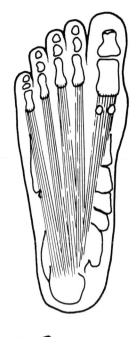

Fig. 3.19 Anatomy of the plantar fascia, divided into five slips which are attached to the bases of the proximal phalanges. At the great toe they embrace the sesamoid bones.

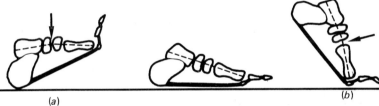

(a)   (b)

Fig. 3.20 (a) The first arch rise at heel contact actively initiated by the long extensors of the toes. (b) Passive arch rise at the end-of-stance phase.

the inner side and there is, in consequence, supination of the foot. As the fore-foot reaches the ground there is a muscle-controlled de-extension with lowering of the arch (Fig. 3.20). This is another shock-absorbing mechanism. With the toe rocker this is repeated passively, converting the foot into a rigid structure to play a part in control of the rise and fall of the body centre of mass. This mechanism is one of the reasons why the shape of the foot is not a static quantity and why an unmodified cast of the foot is not satisfactory in producing footwear.

Abnormal and orthotic-assisted gait uses a selection of these components, or special examples of them, i.e. the transfer of horizontal pelvic rotation to rotating plates beneath the feet in swivel walkers.

PART II CLASSIFICATION OF ORTHOSES

4

Introduction

Classification is a tool in the scientific management of any subject and can be defined as 'a systematic distribution or arrangement in a class or classes'. Nevertheless, it must be approached with caution. Once made, classification tends to take on both an immutability and exclusiveness as though there was nothing more to be said about the group of objects, diseases or persons under consideration. To diminish these dangers, several classifications from different points of view are always advisable and the test of such qualifications is that they should be both a means of understanding and retaining information. In this instance they should also be a tool in the process of clinical decision making, in the design of orthoses and their management in clinical practice.

In orthoses classification can be:

1. Functional (biomechanical)—related to the way in which an orthosis is thought to work.
2. Functional (descriptive)—related to the required criteria for treatment.
3. Ideal characteristics of orthoses. Many are interrelated.
4. Nosological—diseases for which orthoses are used and their function in that disease.
5. Regional—area of the body being treated.

No matter what classification is used it has to be appreciated that:

1. All orthoses have disadvantages in addition to advantages. Awareness of the balance of these is important in prescribing. For example, in the early Milwaukee splint over-enthusiastic usage of distraction with a well-fitting pelvic corset at one end and pressure pads bearing on the mandible at the upper end lead to unacceptable deformities of the lower jaw. Again, the provision of a plastic below-knee splint providing plantar flexion resistance will be an advantage at the beginning of stance but may adversely constrain dorsiflexion at the end.
2. Orthoses commonly have a combination of more than one function.
3. A combination of surgery and orthosis (surgical–orthotic integration) may be required to produce the optimum result. An orthosis must not be prescribed as a substitute for appropriate surgery. This often leads to unrealistic demands being made on the orthosis and the orthotist with poor results.
4. An orthosis can change its functional biomechanical category as a result of experience or research even though based on acceptable mechanical theory when first designed. A classic example of this is the change from passive to the active function with the Milwaukee brace.

5

A functional biomechanical classification

An orthosis:

1. Rests a joint or fracture in a chosen position.
2. Totally or partially relieves stress from a joint or bone, i.e. longitudinal stress relief. Most commonly this is compressive and longitudinal—i.e. weight—but occasionally can be tensional (see Chapter 11) or torsional.
3. Stabilizes a joint or joints in a chosen position, often referred to as a correction of a mobile deformity. The basic principle is to put the part in a normal position so that the major mechanical stresses are within the part, and the forces required to maintain this position are minimal.
4. Corrects, prevents, or supports a fixed or only partially correctable deformity.
5. Exercises muscles and joints.
6. Controls joint range (normal and abnormal) and/or direction during activity.
7. Transmits forces.
8. Re-educates phasic muscle activity.
9. Provides coverage, either cosmetic or protective, or compressive.
10. Compensates for deformity.
11. Reduces heat loss.
12. Acts as a placebo.

These shall now be considered in greater detail.

RESTING A JOINT OR FRACTURE IN A CHOSEN POSITION

In general this can be subdivided into:

1. Orthoses used in bed where the applied forces remain more or less constant in direction, although not necessarily in degree.
2. Those used in an ambulatory patient.

A classic example of the first type is the Thomas Bed Knee Splint. When used as treatment for a fractured femoral shaft, forces combining to produce shortening and angulation are twofold (Fig. 5.1): (a) muscular spasm, causing overlap of the fracture; (b) gravity, causing downward angulation. The latter is usually dealt with by an appropriate arrangement of slings which, if correctly

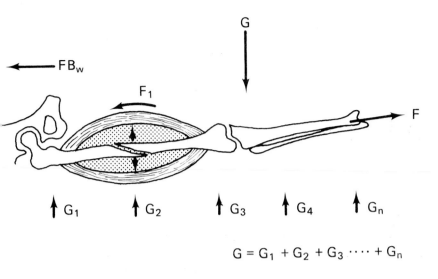

Fig. 5.1 Forces in the production of a state of equilibrium during traction treatment of a fractured femoral shaft. F_1 = muscle contraction. F = traction. FB_W = force from body weight less friction. G = gravity. G_1–G_N = sling reactive support.

adjusted, will each take a share of the load deriving from the weight of the limb. The slings also minimize the interface pressure as the limb changes in contour owing to diminution of swelling and haematoma combined with muscle wastage. It will clearly require readjustment to maintain both the position of the fracture and the optimum interface pressure.

The primary internally generated force derives from muscle spasm of the thigh muscle distended by haematoma. In order to overcome this an equal and opposite reaction must be applied. This can be either sliding or fixed. In sliding, a weight hanging over the end of the bed, independent of the orthosis, provides the necessary force and must be opposed by a force applied to the other end of the leg, traction thereby being localized to the fracture site and not pulling the patient out of bed (Fig. 5.2). This is achieved in practice by friction of the lying patient and body weight with some elevation to the foot of the bed. The disadvantage of this system is that as the haematoma goes down and the muscles waste, the primary force diminishes, and unless the traction force is diminished at the same time distraction of the fracture will occur. This tends to be a rather arbitrary process as the force to be overcome cannot be measured.

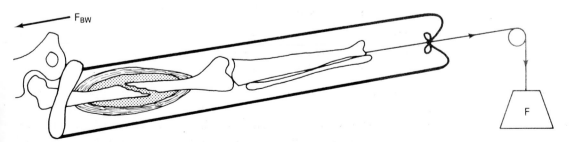

Fig. 5.2 Sliding traction. F_{BW} = force of body weight less friction: F = force of traction weight. F_{BW} = F.

Thomas himself used fixed traction. Here the orthosis is used both for traction and for anti-gravitational support. The advantage of this system is that it is self-regulating. The distal portion of the fracture is connected preferably by skeletal transfixation and a rigid stirrup to a threaded rod passing through a tube with a flynut on the thread distal to the tube which, in turn, has a hook to go over the end of the orthosis (Fig. 5.3). By tightening this nut the traction is applied to the distal end of the fracture, and it is drawn into perfect length. At this moment the force within the system can be determined by a spring balance inserted into a loop conveniently placed on the far end of the threaded rod. It proves to be commonly in the region of 9 kg (20 lb). There will therefore be an equal and opposite reaction to this at the ischial tuberosity against the ring. This high interface pressure can be diminished by raising the foot of the bed. Gravity will produce a force on the pelvis tending to move the pelvis away from the ring; but no movement will occur, and therefore no distraction of the fracture, provided that this force is less than that within the leg system. It is difficult to monitor this objectively, but observation that there is a slight residual interface pressure will confirm that the system has not been converted into sliding traction from the upper end.

As the primary force decreases the length of the femur cannot increase as the system is a rigid one. The force in the system can be monitored daily and

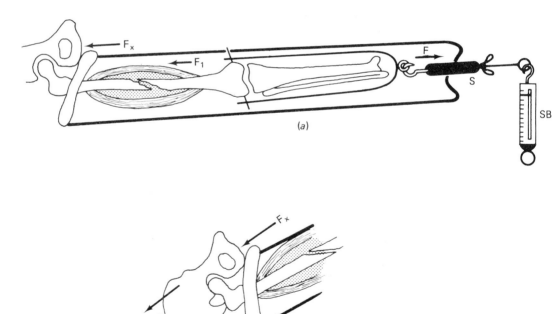

Fig. 5.3 (a) Fixed traction. (b) Diminution of interface pressure. F_x = reaction force against orthotic ring; F_1 = force generated by muscle spasm; F = reaction force against distal end of orthosis; S = screw thread mechanism to achieve length; SB = spring balance; FBW = force of body weight less friction.

as it diminishes the foot of the bed may be lowered to keep interface pressure at the ischial tuberosity still tolerable, at the same time avoiding the institution of a sliding traction from the proximal end which would distract the fracture.

Such a situation is an ideal one, largely self-regulating as regards fracture lengths but capable of being monitored as regards the primary force throughout the period of immobilization. Lateral angulation of the fracture can be controlled by application of the three-point principal, always provided that there is a soft-tissue hinge (Fig. 5.4).

When orthoses (commonly plaster casts or cast braces) are used in the treatment of fractures in patients who are up and about, the situation changes radically in several respects:

1. Movement of the part in space means that the direction of gravitational forces is changing frequently and considerably and cannot be used for fracture control.
2. In addition to some spasm in the early stages, there will be more muscular activity when moving the limb whether weight bearing or not.
3. Dynamic inertial forces are present owing to movement of limb and cast.
4. Where weight bearing occurs the forces within the system are considerably higher. For example, compared with 9 kg (20 lb) compressive force indicated above, forces in a cast brace for a fractured femur could be in the order of 45 kg (100 lb) or more.

This is the basis for the declared orthodoxy in application of plaster casts for treatment of fractures, particularly in the lower limb, namely that the plaster should go, as far as is possible beyond the joints above and below the fracture. Hicks (1960) pointed out that this could, in fact, be a cause of deformity. For example, in a fracture of the mid-shaft of the tibia when the leg was exercised,

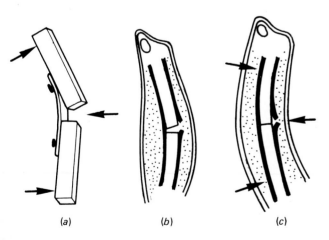

(a)   (b)   (c)

Fig. 5.4 (a) Three-point fixation applied to an articulated structure limited in one direction, for example by a soft-tissue hinge in a fracture or the posterior capsule in the knee joint. (b) Soft-tissue hinge in a fracture treated by a plaster cast. Cast matching the anatomical outline, here in an arm, does not provide satisfactory fixation. (c) Note the necessary discrepancy between normal contour of limb and that of the cast.

muscles inserted around the fracture site would in the intact bone normally be regarded as inserted into the foot and used in the movement of this. Because of the fixation of the foot they exert a reversed action, origin becoming insertion, and the 'new joint' (the fracture) would be moved. Muscle activity within orthoses produces forces which at this time are largely disregarded, quantitatively or qualitatively. In another area of function (the Milwaukee brace) there is good reason to believe that they can be beneficial.

Whatever the mechanical principles used, perfect immobilization of the fracture site will not be obtained. There is reason to suppose that a small amount of motion is beneficial in stimulating union of fractures. In general the following principles can be used for immobilization.

Three-point fixation

When used to control an area of hinge mobility three forces only are required in one plane (Fig. 5.4). Charnley (1950) indicated that in a fracture this 'hinge' consisted of periosteum and attached muscles and was almost always present. Radiographically, it would be on the side away from the opening of the deformed fracture and could be detected during manipulation of a fracture under anaesthesia. Appropriately placed pads would stabilize the 'hinge'—one on the opposite side of the fracture to the hinge and two, one above and one below, placed at the greatest practical distance from it.

The further these forces are apart the smaller the force necessary at each site, the single force being the sum of the other two, which are not necessarily equal but are each inversely proportional to the distance from the articulation. The important practical implication of this is that in applying a plaster cast regard has to be paid to areas of application of the forces. The cast should, therefore, not follow the contours of the normal corresponding limb, but should be somewhat deformed to produce these pressure points, and this is the area where unless appropriate precautions are taken troublesome interface problems will occur. The points should be not only as far as possible from the fracture, but applied over the largest area and appropriately padded.

Hydrodynamic soft-tissue compression (Fig. 5.5)

The use of pneumatic splints for primary first-aid care of fractures has shown that often perfect reduction is obtained by simply applying the orthosis and inflating it. Alas, so often with subsequent orthodox treatment in plaster-of-Paris casts this position is lost. It is interesting to consider how this excellent initial result is achieved—the resultant forces of the uniform compression producing both traction and automatic alignment. It is easier to appreciate this if one considers the displaced fracture causing an increase in bulk of the surrounding area—gently rising compression around this squeezes the ends apart restoring as far as possible the minimum bulk of the leg. Similarly, casts applied firmly—often using elastic plaster bandages initially—will resist deformation of the fracture as loading is applied in the act of walking. This principle is often referred to as total contact. Certainly total contact is the optimum but it is the

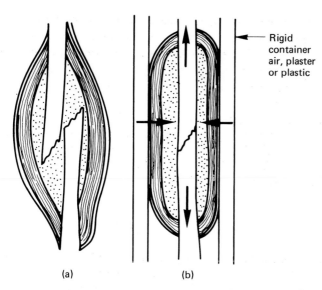

Rigid
container
air, plaster
or plastic

(a)   (b)

Fig. 5.5 Hydrodynamic soft-tissue compression. (a) Overlap of a fresh fracture occurs as a consequence of muscle spasm and the strength of this is increased by extension of the muscle envelope by haematoma. (b) The application of a pneumatic orthosis compresses this area and forces develop as shown which both distract the fracture and by pushing transversely around the circumference re-align it. Because this system works hydrodynamically it can only do so efficiently when the deep fascial envelope containing the muscles and haematoma is intact.

During functional bracing, compressive forces are applied to the fracture as weight bearing is assumed and the possible effects of these, to cause or increase fracture overlap and angulation, are then resisted, in part by the compressed soft tissues as in the pneumatic splint, in part by muscle contraction and partly as a purely mechanical 'anti-buckling' device using three- or four-point fixation.

internal hydrodynamics that provide the beneficial effect (see Functional Bracing, page 165).

TO RELIEVE COMPRESSIVE STRESS TOTALLY OR PARTIALLY (COMMONLY WEIGHT FROM A JOINT OR BONE)

This function is confined mainly to the lower limb, from the hip joint downwards. Where the aim is total relief, in general, an attempt has been made to bypass the limb by transmitting the body weight directly from the pelvis to the floor through an orthosis which may be a crutch or a brace fixed to the limb. It has long been recognized that the ring top caliper is virtually useless in this respect. The small ischial interface area would be required to tolerate a compressive load of about 1.4 × body weight during walking if the ring could be maintained in perfect position. However, no matter how tight the ring is made it is always displaced during activity by the contracting hamstrings attached to the ischial tuberosity which push it medially and upwards into the perineum. The solution to this is not the over-zealous procedure of continually

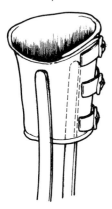

Fig. 5.6 Bucket-top on long leg brace (KAFO).

lengthening the splint to make it well and truly perineal bearing, telling the patient that he will soon get used to it. The perineum is particularly badly designed to bear weight. There are two solutions to this upper-end problem:

1. The bucket-top caliper, when an endeavour is made to obtain some degree of total contact with the soft tissues of the upper thigh (Fig. 5.6).

    or

2. More efficiently, to provide a quadrilateral plastic socket (Fig. 5.7) of the type used in prosthetics, the shape of which has been designed to provide three advantages:

    (a) To distribute weight over the greatest possible area, both at the ischial tuberosity and by firm contact pressure acting on the muscles around the circumference of the thigh, particularly gluteus maximus.

    (b) To prevent displacement of the load from the chosen area during the dynamic changes in limb shape.

    (c) To provide a well-tolerated situation in sitting, a feature noticeably absent from other types of top when applied high up the thigh to try to achieve weight relief. This is achieved by the flat posterior edge.

Used in prosthetics such a socket is made in one piece, but this is not always possible in orthotics. It may be necessary to divide it anteriorly to allow the foot to go through and this will inevitably diminish the efficiency of support even with firm circumferential straps. This inefficiency can be minimized if the two halves interlock with a tongue and metal loop arrangement (Fig. 5.7(b)). Without this when compressive forces are applied, one segment shears downwards in relationship to the other with diminution of fit and contact.

In order to investigate the effectiveness of such devices, experiments have been performed (Lehmann *et al.*, 1970a,b, 1971, 1976) with the orthosis strain gauged and the patient walking on a force platform, the difference between the two results indicating the load through the limb.

Fig. 5.7 Quadrilateral plastic top. Interlocking arrangement on the opening of a quadrilateral socket prevents shearing of one segment in relationship to another under loading and therefore loss of efficient support.

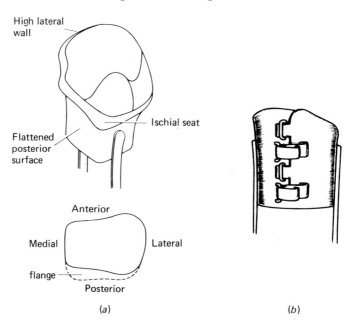

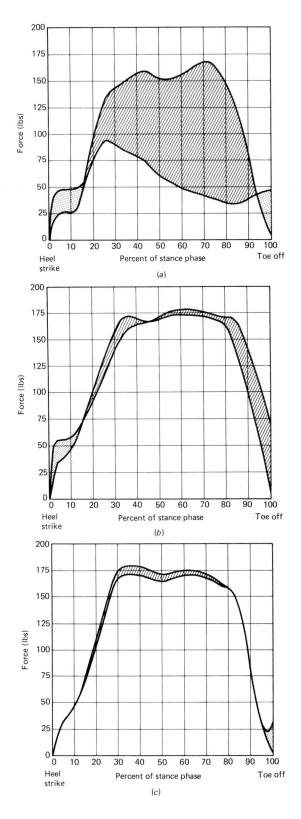

Fig. 5.8 The hatched area represents the difference between the force taken through the long leg brace (KAFO) and that recorded on the force plate. The plain area below these two curves represents the degree of weight-bearing relief. The dotted areas represent a resultant force away from the force plate and this is due to muscular activity within the orthosis. (a) A ring top. (b) A quadrilateral socket with fixed ankle and rocker sole shoe. (c) A patten-ended brace.

With a ring-top caliper there is a very modest reduction in limb loading (Fig. 5.8(a)). It is noted that there are two areas in which the direction of the force within the splint was upwards and electromyography showed this to be due to the action of the plantar flexors of the ankle.

Considerable improvement was achieved by using a quadrilateral socket, reducing the function of the plantar flexors by elevating the anatomical heel 1.5 cm (5/8 in) from the inner surface of the shoe and providing square sockets to restrict the ankle rocker. This last was compensated for by a rigid rocker sole to:

1. Reduce toe contact pressure.
2. Diminish ground reaction forces.

Considerable improvement was achieved (Fig. 5.8(b)). The most efficient instrument, not unexpectedly, was the patten-ended device as shown in Fig. 5.8(c), always provided that it was of adequate length to allow complete suspension of the foot. Patten-ended calipers which provide either a platform for the shoe to rest on or even footdrop stops which are supposed to slide on the side bar but commonly jam, will negate the mechanical advantages and give little better result than an ordinary caliper.

Even with full precautions, the patten-ended device may not necessarily relieve all stress on the hip joint. If in the act of walking abductors of the hip are functioning (Fig. 5.9) they could produce a compressive force on the hip unmonitored in this experiment. In a very small series it has been demonstrated that these muscles do not work during this form of gait. Hence their effects can probably be excluded.

In an endeavour to avoid all these problems weight can be taken entirely from one limb and transferred to a crutch, as in the Snyder sling (Snyder, 1947) (Fig. 5.10). This has the great practical disadvantage that it is totally under control of the patient and is unlikely to be consistently maintained in the majority of cases. A more rigorous solution is the Birmingham Perthes' splint (Fig. 5.11) where in addition to total weight relieving, the hip joint is put in a chosen position, namely abduction and internal rotation, that of so-called maximal containment (Harrison *et al.*, 1969). Control of the splint is removed from the patient by appropriate padlocks. The problem of splintage working on this principle is that in a potentially bilateral condition the question of increased stress on the contralateral hip may arise. Investigation at ORLAU on a force platform showed that used in an orthodox and expected fashion no increase in stress above that normally encountered occurred. The investigation brought to light the hitherto unrealized fact that a number of these patients, quite independently, find that they can progress for short distances efficiently by hopping on the good leg and not using crutches through which the load is normally taken, and do this more commonly. The force on this hip then can rise to six times body weight or more! It highlighted an important element in orthotic design and usage—namely that inspection in a clinic does not provide full usage information.

A similar example was the recurrent breakage of a long leg brace used for knee stabilization by a lightly built young lady. This device had been designed by engineers to have a safety tolerance of three times all predicted forces yet she broke it each week. Only by following the patient was it discovered that she regularly jumped from a moving bus. She regarded this as such a natural feature of her life, that she failed to identify it as a particular or relevant event when questioned closely.

STABILIZING A JOINT OR JOINTS IN A CHOSEN POSITION
(often referred to as correction of a mobile deformity)

'Stabilize' is used here in a strictly mechanical sense and the classic example is the caliper used for the knee with a paralysed quadriceps mechanism.

If such a knee can slightly hyperextend when walking, on a level surface no stabilizing device is in fact required. The leg can be swung forward by action of the hip flexors and the knee will extend inertially. The heel is grounded and because the ground reaction passes in front of the knee joint, extension is maintained without muscular effort. This can be reinforced by action of the hip extensors. Problems arise, however, on rough or irregular ground and particularly on a slope away from the patient when the reactive force in relationship to the knee joint produces a flexion moment at the knee and a stabilizing orthosis is required (see Fig. 3.5, page 24).

Provided the knee fully extends, the load in the leg passes almost entirely through the skeletal structures and the force required at each of the three fixation points used to secure stabilization is very modest, placing minimal stress

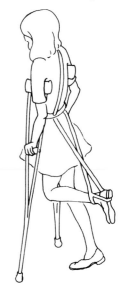

Fig. 5.10 Snyder sling provides total weight relief when worn but is suitable only for unilateral disease. Easy for patient to remove.

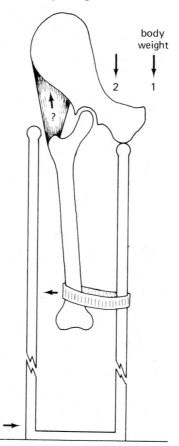

Fig. 5.9 Schematic diagram of the active forces in a patten-ended caliper with possible contraction of the abductors and consequent compression force at the hip joint. 1 is usual line of body weight; 2 is position to which it is automatically moved to avoid need for muscle contraction which would produce hip joint compression.

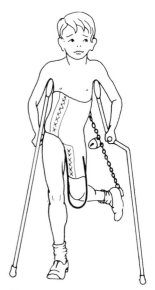

Fig. 5.11 Birmingham splint. This provides total weight relief and optimum containment of the femoral head. Suitable for unilateral disease only. Difficult for the patient to remove.

on the orthosis and the interface. In such circumstances despite poor design and manufacture an orthosis can be very satisfactory to the patient.

The situation alters considerably, however, when there is a flexion contracture of the knee. The classification of the orthosis changes to support of a fixed deformity, because the force required at the fixation points rises steeply, particularly over the front of the knee. The rate of increased moment about the knee compared with degree of flexion is illustrated in Fig. 5.12. The design of the orthosis to resist this is important in regard to length (Fig. 5.13) and the force has then to be distributed over the maximum area to reduce pressure.

High force has two major ill effects:

1. Interface pressure, particularly important in insensitive areas with potential for ulceration.
2. Generation of internal forces which can cause a subluxation of the tibia posteriorly on the femur. The internal resolution of forces (Fig. 5.14) will produce the subluxation if the forward movement of the femur is not resisted. This, therefore, requires a band over the lower femur and it is convenient to join tibial and femoral bands together in orthodox knee pads which prevent divergence of these straps which would otherwise occur because of the resolution forces at the point of contact with the leg. With the straight knee the situation can be controlled without danger by a single strap over the front of the upper tibia and because of the negligible

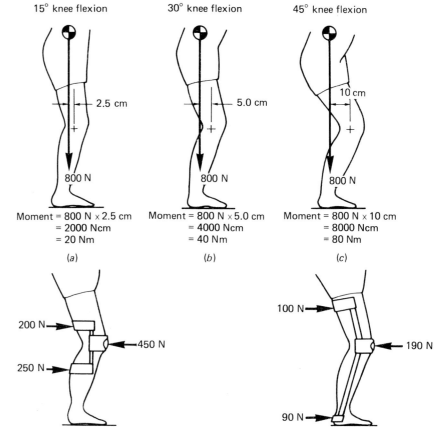

15° knee flexion   30° knee flexion   45° knee flexion

2.5 cm   5.0 cm   10 cm

800 N   800 N   800 N

Moment = 800 N × 2.5 cm   Moment = 800 N × 5.0 cm   Moment = 800 N × 10 cm
= 2000 Ncm   = 4000 Ncm   = 8000 Ncm
= 20 Nm   = 40 Nm   = 80 Nm

(a)   (b)   (c)

Fig. 5.12 The increase in bending moment with increased knee flexion and therefore the increase in force necessary to resist this.

200 N→   ←450 N   100 N→   ←190 N
250 N→   90 N→

Fig. 5.13 The longer the orthosis resisting flexion, the smaller the force applied at each of the three point fixations.

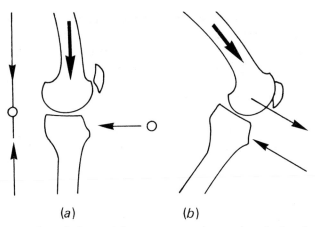

Fig. 5.14 (a) With a straight knee, as no force is required to be applied to the tibia to maintain stability, there is no tendency for the tibio-fibular subluxation which will occur as in (b) due to the resolution of forces.

force a touch and close (Velcro) strap can be used with the elimination of many time-consuming buckles, commonly and unnecessarily provided.

In the adverse situation the ill effects can be reduced by:

1. Surgical intervention to remove the knee contracture.
2. Reduction in the longitudinal loading by a quadrilateral or bucket socket or combined with a lower-end design of the caliper (KAFO) to the heel of the shoe.

A similar situation exists in the grossly pronated foot. If this is mobile it can be restored to the stable position and the forces required to maintain this stability are slight, but in those cases where correction is not possible the device is transformed into a supportive rather than stabilizing device with high interface pressure applied over the inner side of the foot where it cannot be well tolerated. This is an indication for operative correction.

Long leg braces in this class for adults are usually provided with articulations used for sitting. If abnormal stresses are not to be imposed on the anatomical and orthotic joints and also on the interface, reasonable correspondence between the axis of the knee and orthosis must be obtained (see page 156).

CORRECTION, PREVENTION, OR SUPPORT OF A DEFORMITY

Orthoses used to correct a deformity are by far and away the most difficult to design and maintain. The following points must be observed:

1. To be certain that force is applied only to the point of deformity, and does not deform normal tissues, e.g. it is easy to produce deformity of the ribs rather than to correct spinal deformity if this corrective force is not applied to the strongest axis of the rib, namely the longitudinal.
2. To apply the force continuously and maximally consistent with comfort and safety, particularly at the interface contact.

Force can be produced by:

1. Muscular energy to produce active correction.
2. Translation of gravitational energy—passive.
3. Stored energy, usually in some form of spring or torsion device—passive.

Active correction, where possible, has many advantages as the force is always available, whereas in the stored-energy devices once some degree of correction has been obtained the stored energy is lost and constant adjustments are therefore necessary. Large joints are commonly mobilized by muscle activity without the use of orthoses but difficulties may be encountered when the muscles act over a number of joints close together, as for example in stiff interphalangeal joints of the hand. In such circumstances when the metacarpophalangeal joints are mobile, physiotherapy often proves disappointing. The application of an elongated Colles' type of plaster to immobilize the proximal mobile joints, however, will often succeed quite rapidly, because the force is now concentrated at the point required to produce interphalangeal mobility (see Fig. 2.5). Muscle shortening of the triceps surae, for example, will remain whilst the knee and ankle are mobile but once the ankle is fixed in a position of maximum correction, movement of the knee will rapidly, often in a few days, produce elongation of the muscle belly.

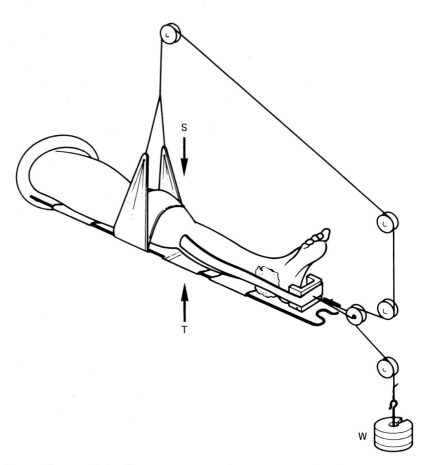

Fig. 5.15 Correction of a knee flexion contracture using Agnes Hunt traction. The pulley system provides longitudinal traction of force 2W and a force (S) pressing down on the knee with a reactive force (T) from a fixed sling pressing upwards against the head of the tibia, tending to reduce any subluxation.

A good example of passive correction using a gravitational translation, and a force therefore continuously acting, is the device designed and used by Dame Agnes Hunt for the correction of the rheumatoid knee (Fig. 5.15). This provides two applied forces to the knee, both traction and extension working simultaneously and maintained continuously as the correction occurs. Because downward forces are applied to the femur with an upwards reactive force to the back of the tibia this represents a reversal of the mechanics of a tibio-femoral subluxation and gives the best chance of a true correction of such a knee.

A transition between passive and active correction is provided by the Milwaukee brace. Initially this was designed to provide three passive correction forces (Fig. 5.16), traction being the most efficient for the marked curve and three-point fixation and turning moments for the smaller curves. Traction applied in this way reacted with the mandible and because, when a force is applied to a normal growing bone and to a deformity, the weaker area will yield, iatrogenic (doctor produced) deformities of the mandible occur and this point of application has now been abandoned. The hyoid mould now provided plays no part in passive traction, and it is now thought that advantage is being taken of the provision by the orthosis of points of reaction for internally generated muscle forces, in a way analogous to the forces applied to the fractured tibia previously indicated. Here the result can be advantageous. The situation is not yet completely defined, yet it is easy to see that extension of the upper cervical spine will press the skull on to the occipital support and so produce active longitudinal traction because this occipital interface is connected via the longitudinal struts to the pelvis.

A conceptual step away from orthotic correction is embodied in the statement 'that correction could only occur where adequate growth potential existed' (Blount and Moe, 1973). This suggested that the forces applied could be less than those required purely for mechanical correction and were designed to influence the biological situation. This is an important concept in all orthoses concerned with children. The problem is that one so designed to

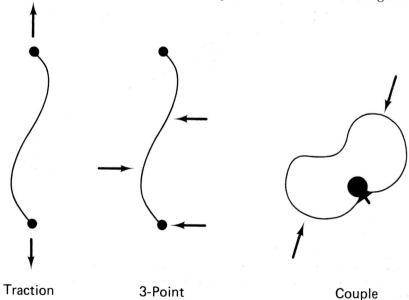

Traction   3-Point   Couple

Fig. 5.16 The three modes of correction in the Milwaukee brace.

influence the growing state could do so adversely, if the point of application is not precisely controlled. It has been suggested, for example, that much of the anteversion seen in congenital dislocation of the hip has been produced in the past by the type of splintage used. Certainly there is very adequate animal experimentation to support this view (Appleton, 1934; Wilkinson, 1962). Caution must, therefore, be expressed in the use of such devices as 'twisters' (Fig. 5.17) for the correction of internal torsion of the legs. These are energy-storage devices, the object of which is to relieve torsion of the legs. No one has produced evidence to determine what force is necessary for this, whether in such devices its effects are limited to bone growth or whether joints can be mal-effected, and no one has shown by controlled observation that the results produced are better than those that occur by normal growth processes. The difficulties of designing such an efficient apparatus are probably the best safeguard against iatrogenic complications.

One other subcategory is important, the avoidance of secondary deformity. For example: the relationship of joint hypermobility in early childhood to late hypermobile flat foot with the tight Achilles tendon must be accepted now as reasonably established, and one knows that this condition can be disabling (Harris and Beath, 1948). It appears theoretically reasonable and therapeutically successful to hold the foot in a corrected position from the time walking commences to avoid the development of secondary deformities, in the main the stretching of the medial capsule of the mid-tarsal joint and to a lesser extent those at the bases of the metatarsal rays. It could be argued that because at this stage deformity is entirely mobile that this is a stabilization process.

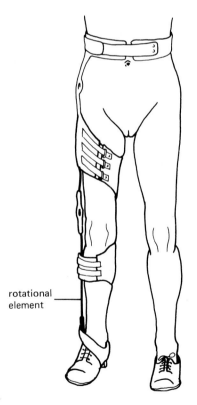

rotational element

Fig. 5.17 'Twister' brace. A potentially corrective force is derived from that stored in the longitudinal rotational element at the time of application. It is commonly a metallic multi-strand cable or a resin-bonded glass fibre.

Certainly this occurs but it can be regarded also as preventative of secondary changes in bone, tendon and joint shape, for once held corrected the condition tends to the normal as hypermobility diminishes, usually at a much slower rate than occurs in normal children.

Another area of this type in which orthoses have been much used in the past was where neurological muscle imbalance exists. Clearly in most of these cases the orthosis is much less efficient in preventing deformity than the muscle imbalance is in causing it, assisted as it often is by growth changes. If, however, orthoses could be designed to eliminate all muscle activity in the affected parts then the ill effects of muscle imbalance might well be kept at bay. Possibly an example of this is the McKibben splint for spina bifida which can succeed apparently if used during the first year of life in maintaining the hip in place despite muscle imbalance because it removes or diminishes all muscle activity (Fig. 5.18). It is contended that following this the hip will tend to remain stable without further treatment. In general, however, the presence of muscle imbalance is a clear indication for surgical intervention in addition to or in place of orthotic treatment.

The classic example of passive stretching by means of stored energy is embodied on some occasions in the multi-functional so-called 'lively splints' used for the upper limb (Fig. 5.19) and generally used to try to improve the range of joint mobility limited by intra- and extra-articular contractures without at the same time losing another range of joint movement. Increased flexion of interphalangeal joints in the fingers may be a valuable functional gain always provided that extension is maintained. Energy is stored in various types of springs or elastic, the former relying on both structure and material storage capacity and the latter on material, and as the capacity varies in respect of shape and length this will alter as the deformity is corrected, and requires corresponding modification of the orthosis. The primary energy for storage comes, of course, from the muscles of the other hand when the device is put on and may then be supplemented by such activities as are available in the flexor muscles. In this type of splintage the point of application and interface pressure also needs constant monitoring, particularly as such problems are commonly associated with nerve and/or muscular damage.

An interesting variant of the situation occurs in wedged plasters for deformity as in the Kite club foot plaster. A well-fitting plaster is applied to the

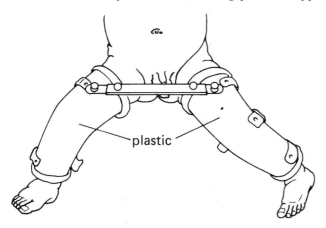

Fig. 5.18 McKibben's splint used in spina bifida for correcting a dislocating hip on the left side which is held abducted and internally rotated.

deformed foot. When dry it is divided for two-thirds of its diameter in a line which runs through the axis of the joint to be stretched. The plaster is then vigorously stretched open and replastered in the position (Fig. 5.20). At this time energy is loading into the elastic structures of the deformed limb and yielding of these is relied upon for correction. It is possible, in these circumstances, that the energy is stored for only a matter of hours so that frequent changes are compatible with the most efficient correction.

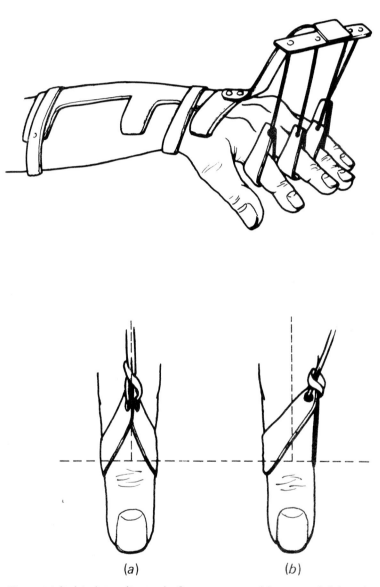

(a)   (b)

Fig. 5.19 A 'lively' splint used to stretch a flexion contracture of the metacarpal-phalangeal (mcp) joints. Note that the applied force is at right angles to the phalanges (a) to achieve the most efficient moment about the mcp joints and that its application is limited to these joints. The line of application of force must be at right angles to the axis of the joint if a secondary deformity is to be avoided, and *not* as in (b).

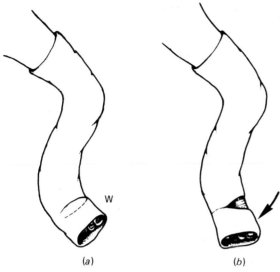

Fig. 5.20 The kite club-foot plaster. (a) Wedge cut W. (b) Wedge opened.

EXERCISE OF MUSCLES AND JOINTS

In practice this is the commonest and most consistent function of the upper limb 'lively splints'. Again energy is stored in various flexible devices employing combinations of a range of components including articulations, springs and elastic. In this case, however, they are loaded by primary energy from the muscles of the same limb and the act of doing this exercises and strengthens muscles and keeps joints mobile. Stored energy is then released as a substitute for missing motors in paralytic conditions.

CONTROL OF JOINT RANGE AND/OR DIRECTION DURING ACTIVITY

A common example of this is the range of devices used to prevent foot drop. As these function during the swing phase, they are not stabilizing devices when used in the uncomplicated paralytic condition with full joint mobility but prevent plantar flexion beyond 5 degrees to allow the normal degree of foot clearance in this phase if the control of the other joints is normal. Such patients without orthoses use an increased knee and hip flexion to reduce the overall relative lengthening of the leg with the dropped foot and in such circumstance the orthosis is in part cosmetic as well as reducing energy expenditure. Where knee and hip control is not normal, provision of such a device becomes functionally more important.

Excessive dorsi-flexion positioning in such an apparatus has the disadvantageous effect of geometrically lengthening the leg. If the patient does not clear the floor the increased orthotic dorsi-flexion often demanded by patients and therapists will be of no avail, and should be resisted. In addition rapid movement of the tibial shank occurs from heel strike to flat foot (Fig. 5.21). If there is

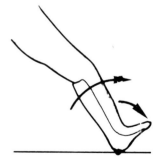

Fig. 5.21 Where plantar flexion of the ankle is resisted, the first half of the ankle rocker function is lost. As the foot goes from heel strike to foot flat the shank is rotated forward, flexing the knee which cannot be tolerated if the quadriceps is paralysed.

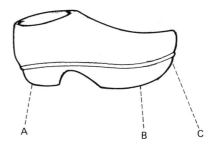

A   B   C

Fig. 5.22 With a plantar resist or fixed ankle AFO, the imposed problems on the shank can be mitigated by an appropriate curved sole contour. The radius of the curve from A to B is an axis at the hip joint, but from B to C the axis is one at the knee joint and the curve is therefore increased. The relatively forward point of this change in axis should be noted.

an associated weakness of knee extensors this may force the knee into flexion (previously avoided by the patient to stabilize this joint) and the overall effect is a considerable reduction in confidence. If for any reason this position cannot be avoided it is possible to mitigate it to some extent by shoe sole alterations (Fig. 5.22).

In foot drop alone the force to be resisted during the stance phase is the weight of the foot. The degree of plantar flexion resist can be made relatively weak which means that the dorsi-flexion resist encountered during late-stance phase can also be weak and the interference with this phase minimized. Where foot drop is associated with spasm or contracture of the triceps surae for example, the situation is more difficult and in extreme degrees problems of maintaining contact between the orthosis and the limb combined with intolerable interface pressure can produce insoluble orthotic problems which require some surgical intervention, often quite simple, such as complete tenotomy of the Achilles tendon under local anaesthetic in order to produce optimum orthotic function.

This is a relatively simple theoretical problem, but if one considers the question of providing bipedal ambulation in the flaccid paraplegic the failure to identify the necessary components of locomotion and gait is widely reflected in the almost universal rejection of such devices in the adult and the eventual rejection in the young.

In general, the theoretical approach to this problem has been to provide stabilization of the knees by long leg bracing and of the hips by use of crutches to prevent flexion collapse. Because the hips are polyaxial four types of problem occur when ambulation is attempted:

1. Forward flexion collapse at the hips, well controlled by crutches (Fig. 5.23(a)).
2. Passive scissoring (Fig. 5.23(b)). If a body posture is assumed in which the hips are ahead of the feet, whether the hips are extended or flexed, one leg will move forward under the influence of gravity if it can be raised from contact with the ground (see Fig. 3.12, page 27). This can be initiated by downward pressure on the ipsilateral crutch and as the swing leg tends to

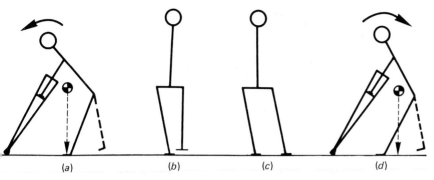

Fig. 5.23 Paraplegic patient walking with crutches and KAFOs. (a) Forward flexion at the hips assisted by the crutches. (b) During one-leg stance the swing leg tends to fall toward or in front of the stance leg. (c) 'Windswept' fall-out during double stance. (d) If the centre of mass comes behind the support leg posterior fall-out occurs which cannot be controlled by crutches.

move forward it will also move inwards to maintain the vertical position in relationship with the ground which gravity imposes whilst the contralateral hip tends to go into adduction, since it lacks abductors. This means that when the swing foot is grounded it will lie either ahead or even lateral to the line of the stance foot so that when the process is repeated the second foot will go behind or rub against the first, either bringing ambulation to a standstill or reducing its efficiency.

3. 'Windswept' fall-out (Fig. 5.23(c)). This is a tendency when both feet are on the ground for one hip to abduct and the other to adduct. Actual falling is more or less controllable by the crutches depending on flexibility, abnormal or otherwise, of the spine and its available muscular control.

4. Posterior fall-out. Whilst the other problems can to some extent be tolerated, albeit with marked reduction in gait efficiency and increased energy cost, posterior fall-out is quite disastrous as it cannot be corrected by the patient. It will occur when the stance leg is forward and the swing leg is first lifted from the ground. If at this time the centre of mass of the whole system—patient, orthoses and crutches—is behind the stance leg there will be a posterior moment about this foot and the patient will either fall backwards or revert to the original stance prior to the elevation of the swing leg with ambulation brought to a standstill (Fig. 5.23(d)).

In considering the orthotic solutions in regard to a new patient one must have a complete knowledge of the neurological situation particularly as in the patchy lesions of spina bifida, motor and sensory paralysis can occur in the legs with some residual joint proprioception. If this exists then the patient can often position his body in space so as to avoid these problems and it is this rather rare type of case in adult traumatic paraplegia who does find useful the usual calipers and crutches supplied.

If this does not exist then orthotic control must be provided and the first requirement is articulations that move as freely as possible and apply minimum constraints in movement occurring under the influence of gravity. This is a question of engineering design and the provision of ball-bearing articulations. The second requirement is that the device should be rigid, or in biochemical terms stiff. Commonly those provided with pelvic bands or thoracic brace are so flexible that they exert minimal control over (2) and (3) and in addition fail in another very important respect, i.e. the control of adduction in one hip when the contralateral leg is raised from the ground. This is a question of efficient energy expenditure and reproduction of the normal dynamic extrinsic stability used in walking is the objective. In the orthotic situation the stance leg which optimally moves forward under the influence of gravity moves again during the interval before the foot returns to the ground under the influence of potential energy. If, however, the contralateral hip adducts, the centre of mass will not only go over the support foot but beyond it; and unless a second injection of energy is provided through the crutch on that side the patient will fall over laterally. Clearly, stability in this situation results in two phases of crutch-conveyed energy expenditure instead of the one which is optimum (see Fig. 3.11, page 26).

Whilst the swing leg is going forward, simultaneous movement is occurring in the stance leg and at this time the orthosis must be used not for control of movement but for transmission of force from the arms through the crutches to a point of reaction on the ground in order to help the patient over the uphill segment (Fig. 5.24).

Posterior fall-out is dealt with by limiting flexion of the hips, a fact that is not easy to appreciate at first sight, but which depends on a complex geometrical relationship between this angle and the length of the crutch. This is in turn related to the desired cosmetic result of relatively vertical posture but much more importantly to the mechanical advantage of the muscles working between the trunk and the arms. These hips are considerably flexed with short crutches as shown in Fig. 5.25(a). The centre of mass will be well forward of the support foot but the posture is near horizontal and when the muscles between trunk and arm contract the efficiency in surmounting the uphill phase is very poor indeed. In Fig. 5.25(b), on the other hand, this problem is overcome but the centre of mass is now behind the support foot (the swing leg being raised) and the patient will fall backwards. The resultant moment about the stance foot is such that there is no reaction at the crutch tips and the

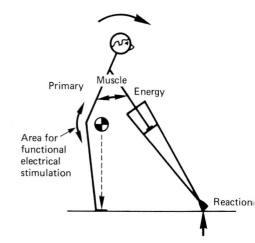

Fig. 5.24 Transmission of force from the arm to the crutches to help the patient over the uphill segment. Experimentally this can be reinforced by stimulation of the extensor muscles of the hip.

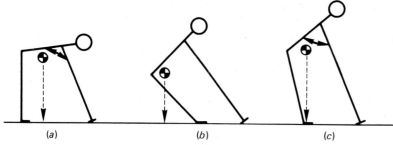

Fig. 5.25 (a) If the hips are considerably flexed to achieve stability short crutches are necessary if the situation in (b) is not to occur. This produces an unacceptable posture and reduces the efficiency of the arm–trunk muscles in moving the body forward. (c) An acceptable position.

patient cannot therefore exert any corrective force. In these circumstances hooks on the end of the crutches would be required.

Optimum flexion of the hips is, therefore, of vital importance if maximum step length is to be achieved with security and propulsion. In practice this is in the region of 10 degrees but may require some modification depending on the available geometry. So critical is this that an assured vigorous walker became immobile when the wear on the limiting stops of his hip articulation became worn to the degree shown in Fig. 5.26. It points also to the fact that these stops need to be made of suitably wear-resistant materials.

Patients initially supplied with this orthosis, known as the Hip Guidance Orthosis (see page 186), commonly find that at first they can only progress using a rollator and not crutches. This is because the rollator, the back legs of which tend to be behind the support foot during this critical phase, provides an increased support area. Gaining confidence, and with training, some patients will then proceed to crutches, the best type of which are 'Canadian

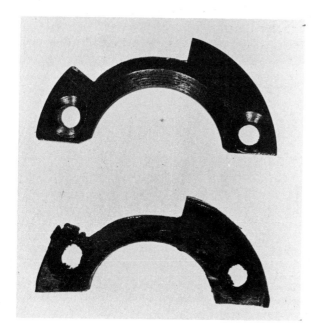

Fig. 5.26 Hip flexion stops used in walking. The amount of wear shown was sufficient to affect the geometry of Fig. 5.25 so as to make independent walking impossible. In consequence, specially strengthened stops were used.

crutches' (Stallard *et al.*, 1978b; Dounis *et al.*, 1980) but where this cannot be achieved consideration of the theoretical situation suggested that improvement might occur if the centre of mass could be brought forward by adding weight to the crutches at the optimum point, i.e. as distally as possible. This has indeed shown to be the case and is an interesting example of the fact that blind adherence to the concept that reduction in the weight of orthoses will necessarily produce improvement in function is not true, and that as in lower-limb prosthetics, the placement of the centre of mass of the limb or the body may be equally important.

There is one further important theoretical consideration in regard to the provision of bipedal gait. Theoretically the foot can be raised from the ground either by abduction of the other hip through an appropriate hinge (limited in adduction to prevent scissoring) or by lateral rotation about the foot/floor contact area, an appropriate shape of the foot sole being provided. Consideration of the geometry here shows that for an equal clearance the former requires the centre of mass to be lifted approximately three times higher compared with the latter (Fig. 5.27) which is therefore to be preferred primarily because of the reduction in energy cost but also because in practice, abduction hinges of the present design rapidly become bound. Furthermore for the sake of rigidity all possible hinges need to be avoided.

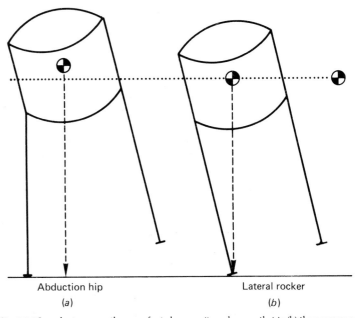

Abduction hip   Lateral rocker

(a)   (b)

Fig. 5.27 In order to secure the same foot clearance it can be seen that in (b) the necessary elevation of the centre of mass, although not marked on this diagram, is significantly less in regard to energy expenditure.

TRANSMISSION OF FORCES

In the previous section it will be noted that there is an overlap between this function and that of control of joint movement providing the mechanical context for the transmission of forces from the arm through the crutches to produce a ground reaction and through the trunk to produce the necessary extension of the hip joint in stance phase for the uphill phase. The potential energy accumulated during this activity becomes kinetic energy during the downhill movement and this is carried forward into the next contralateral stance phase inertially. Because of this, total energy expenditure for such patients can be shown by dynamic gait studies to be very low when walking on the level and to be tolerated although increased when walking up a gradient of one in ten. Lack of rigidity means that some of the energy will be lost in flexing the structure with consequent reduction in efficiency.

Simpler examples of transmission of force are found in upper-limb orthoses. For widespread paralysis of the arm in brachial plexus injury, exoskeletons have been provided. A primary force, from the shoulder for example, or stored energy in the form of compressed gas, transmitted by various linkages (sometimes flexible, such as a bowden cable), is provided for limited functions such as elbow flexion or even simple hand grasp. These devices have a number of quite considerable problems. External power at this time is limited by the power–weight ratio and in general the powerpack is too heavy to be reasonably carried or if light, as in the case of pneumatic cylinders, will function for a relatively short time and requires a large number of available spare refills.

In addition, because of their inevitable complexity, such orthoses require frequent maintenance which can be done only in a relatively sophisticated workshop. The design tendency is in fact to greater complexity, as it is now appreciated that positional feedback and servo-control of the energy supplies is vitally important for their satisfactory function. These factors limit their supply to the severely handicapped for whom in some circumstances they can be invaluable, as for example in some tetraplegic or severe poliomyelitic patients but need careful matching to the individual problem and must have patient acceptance.

An excellent example of the intrinsically powered device is the wrist-driven flexor hinge orthosis (Bisgrove, 1964; Nichols *et al.*, 1978) which translates active wrist extension to interphalangeal flexion of the fingers and extension at the metacarpo-phalangeal joints to provide active prehension (Fig. 5.28).

RE-EDUCATION OF PHASIC MUSCLE ACTIVITY

A very simple example of this occurs in what has been designated in my clinics as the 'nine–ten syndrome'. Children of about this age with high arched feet and a considerable shift of the intermalleolar diameter medially related to their foot support area, who have had no trouble with their feet and indeed have none now, are brought because they have within the last 12 months started to deform and wear their shoes rapidly under the medial aspect of the sole and heel with a gross inwards deformity of the upper. Shoes may become useless within 3 weeks and the condition is a considerable financial burden for the parents.

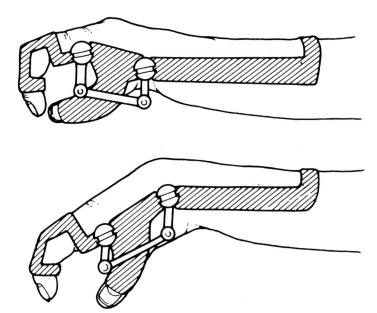

Fig. 5.28 Wrist-driven flexor hinge orthosis. Power is provided by wrist extensors; when the wrist is flexed by gravity the pinch-chuck grip occurs between thumb, index and middle finger-tips and this is opened by using the wrist extensor.

The provision of Rose–Schwartz menisci (see Fig. 13.9) will almost inevitably produce an immediate return to normal shoe wear. After about 1 year these can be abandoned, without recurrence of the syndrome, yet the most careful examination of the foot and leg will reveal no change. One can only conclude that during this period some re-education of the phasic activity of muscles during gait has occurred and once established this habit is permanent.

Much less successful is the endeavour to re-educate phasic muscle activity in cerebral palsy. In patients suffering from muscular malfunction not associated with joint or muscle contractures, a hip orthosis providing a lumbo-thoracic brace articulated through low friction articulations to thigh cuffs will control scissoring if adequately rigid and yet allow reciprocal gait. In patients with an excessive hip and knee flexion producing a gross 'high stepping gait' springs can be incorporated posterially into such articulation with advantage and it is convenient to put these on small outriggers and to make them variable in tension.

Such an orthosis also comes within the category of control of joint movement but in some cases, and these are unfortunately rare, re-educational improvements can occur to some extent. The practical implication of this situation is that objective recording of early gait should be made with video-film and from time to time compared not only with the gait whilst in the apparatus but also without it.

PROVISION OF COVERAGE, EITHER COSMETIC, PROTECTIVE OR COMPRESSIVE

Cosmetic coverage has become easily available with the development of plastics, and a useful example is the provision of an artificial muscle mass to restore the calf muscle outline in certain neurological conditions. Where a plastic drop foot appliance of the contoured type is provided this can be conveniently added. In the same category are the many varieties of replacement required after mastectomy. Although strictly prostheses they are commonly dealt with by specialist orthotists. The advantages of plastic technology have resulted in considerable advances and in general there are now four types depending on the filling—granular, oil, fluid/air and silicone, but in this area the multiplicity of problems and options requires very expert fitting.

In the provision of shoes the cosmetic effect is mainly a negative one. The demand of some patients to have a smaller outside than inside produces an insoluble problem! Nevertheless, within the limits of medical requirements, attention to styling and ornamentation can produce greater acceptability.

Shoes also have a protective function and this is normally related to two forms of mechanical stress—pressure and shear. The problems can be considered in two areas:

1. Encasement—those of foot coverage which could be avoided theoretically by going barefooted.
2. Inevitable—those related to the weightbearing area of the foot, usually the sole, which cannot be avoided in ambulation.

Encasement

Comment will be made on the relationship of the footwear last to the standing shape of the foot and the need to modify this (page 140). In walking changes also occur in the shape of the footwear, and particularly during the 'toe rocker' phase.

This latter causes creasing of the shoe with change in the internal shape at this level if the shoe is flexible. It has been noted recently that some synthetic materials produce harder, sharper internal creases than does leather with consequent increase in adverse effects. Where forefoot deformity diminishes the tolerance to internal creasing, this can be prevented by the provision of a rigid rocker sole. Shoe styling, stitching or overlap may influence the position of these creases adversely. Failure to appreciate this type of change may lead to the prescription of an insole with a rigid toe block to fill the front area of the shoe after amputation of toes. Changes in position of this in various phases of gait (Fig. 5.29) can cause considerable discomfort. In fact, the easiest practical solution to this problem is to allow the patient to pack the toe with cotton wool, which they soon adjust to optimum function and comfort.

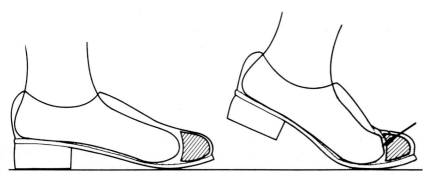

Fig. 5.29 Changes in footwear shape during gait can cause forefoot problems, as in this case where a rigid toe block on an insole has been provided to fill the front area of the shoe after amputation of toes.

Inevitable pressure

This becomes pathological when high-pressure points are present in the sole and the commonest of these are under the metatarsal heads, an area that is normally designed to accommodate pressure with a modified fibro-fatty subcutaneous layer, plantar fascia and thick skin. As a result of continuous pressure the subcutaneous tissue becomes thinned and the skin calloused with local pain. The classic solution is to relieve pressure on this area by providing a raised dome or foam bar behind the metatarsal head which translates the pressure to areas less well adapted to weight bearing and which may include intrinsic muscle. If used for prolonged periods these structures become thinned, a higher dome is then required and eventually no localized relief of this kind can be successful. Such devices, therefore, should not be used except where the cause of pain or pressure in the forefoot is likely to be of short duration. It is more feasible to try to increase the area of applied load substantially and therefore decrease pressure by providing, for example, a moulded insole which can now be easily made of thermoplastic discrete celled plastic foam.

However, this must be used rationally. Where there are prominent areas in the sole these will depress and compress the foam and may indeed completely obliterate any cellular structure, leaving appreciable pressure in the affected areas. Ideally, therefore, a cast of the weight-bearing surface of the foot should be made in relatively thick foam so that no 'bottoming out' occurs. This foam should then be ground down on the flat surface until it just approaches the deepest contour and the removed material replaced by an undeformed layer of foam of about 6 mm (1/4 in). A decision then has to be taken whether the resultant insole can be accommodated in a normal shoe or whether increased depth is required.

In the worst problems encountered, trophic ulceration of neurological conditions such as leprosy, diabetes or spina bifida, particularly where there is ulceration or the scarring of healed ulceration, scrupulous attention to redistribution of pressure can prove disappointing if the presence of shear stress is not recognized and dealt with. There exists at the heel and the metatarsal heads contact articulations which present in general spherical surfaces which can roll either fore or aft or side and do this within the subcutaneous tissue, the skin below remaining relatively unmoving compared with the contact area. When, therefore, the foot passes from the flat foot phase to the toe off the metatarsal heads roll forward relative to the skin (see Fig. 2.6, page 15) and this is a shear absorbing mechanism.

If, however, the subcutaneous tissue is scarred or significantly thinned, internal shear stresses will cause continuing pain or damage. There is only one way in which this can be satisfactorily removed, namely to transfer the rolling mechanism to the shoe contact area. This is done by providing a rigid sole, and it must be absolutely rigid, with an appropriate rocker shape (see Fig. 5.30). In severe conditions it is mandatory to provide, in addition to the pressure-relieving insole described, a wooden or rigid plastic rocker sole to which this is stuck (Fig. 5.30), the whole thing incorporated in an appropriate deep, usually custom-built shoe.

It is convenient at this point to comment on the metatarsal bar, which again must be mounted on a rigid sole if it is not to be pressed into the sole and pro-

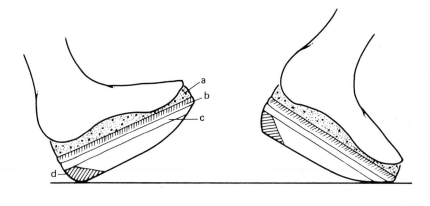

Fig. 5.30 Two layer thermo-plastic foam conforming to the weight-bearing under-surface of the foot with the addition of a wooden or plastic stiffener. The shoe is then made to measure. (a) Deformed foam. (b) Undeformed foam. (c) Solid plate—wood or plastic. (d) Cushion heel.

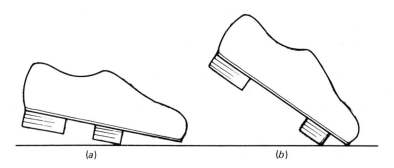

Fig. 5.31 Depending on placement of the metatarsal bar the permitted angle of heel raise without toe extension is varied. From this point of view the forward-placed fulcrum as in (b) is the better one.

duce a corresponding deformation of the inner side of the shoe. It has been customary to place the metatarsal bar far back on the sole. As the purpose of this is to prevent extension of the toes, in theory the further forward the bar the greater the permitted angle of toe rocking without ground reaction causing toe extension (Fig. 5.31). In practice, therefore, the metatarsal bar should be under the metatarsal heads. The present orthodoxy produces an almost functionless bar consequent upon placement and the failure to provide adequate sole rigidity. A rocker sole should also have the area of maximum depth in this region for the same reason and because it reproduces externally the normal 'toe rocker'. If either rocker sole or metatarsal bar is provided this will cause a change in the relationship between sole and heel height and compensatory re-adjustment of the heel height will be necessary, particularly if there is a tight Achilles tendon.

Protective coverage

Protective-helmet orthoses are much used in cerebral palsy and spina bifida. Various forms of these have been designed and the most attractive are often commercially produced replicas of various helmets such as those used on building sites with suitable additional internal padding.

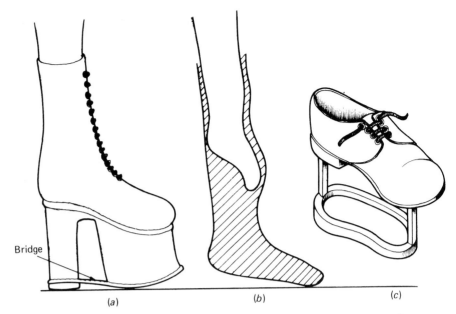

Fig. 5.32 Various ways of compensating for a marked shortening of the leg. (a) An external raise made either of cork or modern rigid plastic foam, encased in leather to give strength. With such a raise a boot is necessary to avoid ankle instability and note should be taken of the bridging leather between the heel and the sole. If this were not in position a divergence of the heel occurs with destruction of the raise. Note the sole contour. The chief complaint of patients wearing any form of raise is the rigidity this imposes on their toe rocker and it has, therefore, to be externalized. (b) The O'Connor extension. A foot-shaped extension to the leg with the ankle in as much equinus as is possible. This requires at least 15 cm (6 in) of shortening to permit prescription. (c) Patten end. This can be useful, particularly in considerable shortening in situations where cosmesis is not important and lightness an advantage.

COMPENSATION FOR DEFORMITY

The simplest example of this is the raise supplied to footwear to compensate for the shortened leg. It is in this area where some meeting place commonly occurs between prostheses and orthoses. The O'Connor extension (Fig. 5.32), for example commonly regarded as an orthosis as it is not used with amputation, is in fact a replacement of or compensation for the missing leg length. Something close to the normal appearance of the leg shank is achieved by placing the foot in maximum equinus and encasing this in a more or less tubular packet attached to an artificial foot which can then be put into a normal shoe.

REDUCTION OF HEAT LOSS

In general where a heat problem exists with orthoses it is that of avoiding excessive production of heat, sometimes called calefaction. However, it has been demonstrated that—particularly in the aged supplied with lumbosacral supports—the only common factor amongst satisfactory appliances has been the quality of heat insulation and this aspect must not be overlooked in the prescription of such devices (Dixon *et al.*, 1972).

ACTION AS A PLACEBO

In orthotic practice a number of patients will be encountered wearing what are clearly totally ineffective devices and one has met patients wearing a Thomas back support provided in childhood 20 years earlier and on one occasion upside down, yet it proved impossible to ween the patient from it. There must be many similar, less obvious and gross examples, where an orthosis plays an appropriate part, defensive or aggressive in the family dynamics. At a regional clinic set up to review all patients who were wearing traditional calipers, to be assessed for providing new cosmetic calipers, the clinical team were surprised that some patients were not willing even to try the more modern development.

It came as a surprise to all when one patient admitted that he was much happier with his clanking old caliper, because when he boarded a bus fellow passengers would immediately be aware of his disability and treat him with compassion. The new type of orthosis was not so visible or audible and consequently did not elicit the same response. In this case the orthosis was used as a psychological persuader.

6

A functional descriptive classification

A major problem in orthotics is that of prescription writing. Prior to the National Health Service the prescriber's requirements were usually given personally to a man who would both fit and manufacture the orthosis. This is now a privilege available to relatively few; and it must be recognized that this will and must remain so, in the interest of optimum standards of orthotic supply. The inevitable consequence of the longer impersonal lines of communication is the necessity to combine in one document the functional defects of the patient with an unambiguous description of the orthosis required. This has been the task to which the American Academy of Orthopaedic Surgeons has applied great skill and perserverance to produce their Biomechanical Analysis systems to serve not only as a bridge of communication between prescriber and orthotist but also to provide valuable information to the therapist and engineer.

It consists of three sections:

1. Description of the patient impairment in functional terms.
2. Treatment objectives.
3. Orthotic recommendations.

DESCRIPTION OF THE PATIENT IMPAIRMENT IN FUNCTIONAL TERMS

This includes the following:

1. Skeletal—bone and joint.
2. Neurological—sensory and motor.
3. Pain.
4. Balance.
5. Skin state.
6. Gait deviations.
7. Other pathology.

Motion is described either as translatory or rotational, where translation means lineal motion either straight or curved; and rotational, motion about a single axis. Combinations can also occur.

This is followed by a summary of functional disability.

TREATMENT OBJECTIVES

These are:

1. Prevention or correction of deformity.
2. Reduction of axial load.
3. Protection of joints.
4. Improvement of ambulation.
5. Treatment of fractures.
6. Other.

ORTHOTIC RECOMMENDATIONS

The extent of the orthosis

This is described by the joints over which the orthosis passes. The body is divided into three segments (Table 6.1). For hand and foot the symbols MP, PIP, DIP are added and for the thumb CM, MP, and IP. In combining these letters the United Nations usage is adopted, i.e. AFO not A.F.O. For those speaking Anglo-Saxon variants, this sometimes results in acceptable acronymic words such as KAFO for the long leg brace. In other areas the result is not so easily acceptable; for example, a Milwaukee brace is CTLSO (cervical thoracic–lumbar sacro-iliac orthosis) and requires 28 control symbols (Harris, 1973). In such cases much time is saved by using the eponym (which strictly speaking derives from the name of a person but commonly is now used for place of origin), always provided that the eponym has a precise and universally accepted meaning. This section is the least important of the three but the convenient acronymic words are becoming part of the international language of orthotics.

Table 6.1   Division of the body for describing the extent of orthoses

Upper limb	Lower limb	Spine
S = shoulder	H = hip	C = cervical
E = elbow	K = knee	T = thoracic
W = wrist	A = ankle	L = lumbar
H = hand	F = foot	SI = sacro-iliac

Control of designated function of joints or articulations

The symbols used are as follows:

F = Free movement.
A = Assist—application of external force to increase range, velocity or force.
R = Resist—application of external force to decrease velocity, range or force.
S = Stop—inclusion of a static unit to avoid undesired motion in one direction. When used alone it means restraint of gross movement in neutral position of joint.

V = Variable—an adjustable unit not requiring structural change. Commonly used with 'stop'.

H = Hold—elimination of all motion in one plane; the position must be specified.

L = Lock—optional lock.

Standard forms have been provided to cover this information which includes diagrams of the skeleton on which joint ranges can be conveniently marked, as can the degree of volitional and hypertonic force (Figs. 6.1–6.3).

This form, although time consuming (even with flexible use of the system outlined in Table 6.1) undoubtedly represents a considerable advance in prescription. For the prescriber who is inclined to feel dissatisfied with the supply situation, to be able to supply this or equivalent information is the first move to improvement. Doing so concentrates the mind wonderfully on defining objectives and expectations as it will if used by the orthotist. Manufacturers require considerable persuading as they are not always as aware of its potential value and it does, if adopted, have a profound influence on manufacturing methods—albeit highly beneficial.

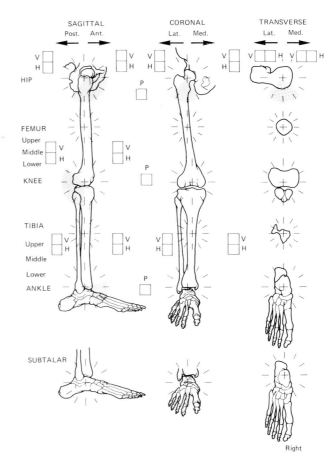

Fig. 6.1 Functional descriptive classification: diagrams for lower limb.

TECHNICAL ANALYSIS FORM   **LOWER LIMB**

Name_____ No._____ Age _____ Sex_____

Date of Onset_____ Cause_____

Occupation _____ Present Lower-Limb Equipment_____

Diagnosis _____
_____
_____

Ambulatory ☐   Non-Ambulatory☐

MAJOR IMPAIRMENTS:
A.   Skeletal
   1.   Bone and Joints: Normal ☐   Abnormal_____
   2.   Ligaments: Normal ☐   Abnormal ☐   Knee: AC ☐   PC ☐   MC ☐   LC ☐
                                       Ankle: MC ☐   LC ☐

   3.   Extremity Shortening: None ☐   Left ☐   Right ☐
       Amount of Discrepancy: A.S.S.-Heel_____   A.S.S.-MTP_____   MTP-Heel_____

B.   Sensation: Normal ☐   Abnormal ☐
   1.   Anaesthesia ☐   Hypaesthesia ☐   Location:_____
      Protective Sensation: Retained ☐   Lost ☐
   2.   Pain ☐   Location:_____

C.   Skin: Normal ☐   Abnormal:_____

D.   Vascular: Normal ☐   Abnormal ☐   Right ☐   Left ☐

E.   Balance: Normal ☐   Impaired ☐   Support:_____

F.   Gait Deviations:_____
    _____

G.   Other Impairments:_____

———————————— **LEGEND** ————————————

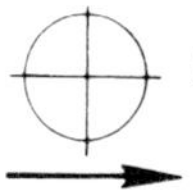

= Direction of Translatory Motion

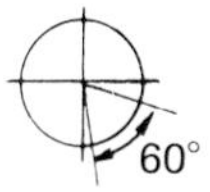

= Abnormal Degree of Rotary Motion   60°

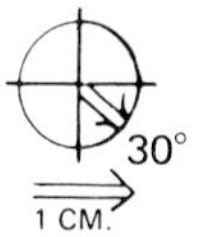

= Fixed Position   30°

1 CM.

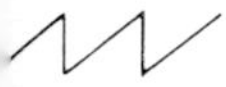

= Fracture

Volitional Force (V)
N = Normal
G = Good
F = Fair
P = Poor
T = Trace
Z = Zero

Hypertonic Muscle (H)
N = Normal
M = Mild
Mo = Moderate
S = Severe

Proprioception (P)
N = Normal
I = Impaired
A = Absent

D = Local Distension or Enlargement

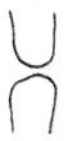

= Pseudarthrosis

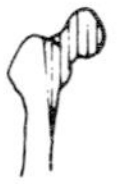

= Absence of Segment

Fig. 6.2 Functional descriptive classification: technical analysis form for lower limb.

Summary of Functional Disability _____

_____

_____

_____

_____

_____

Treatment Objectives:

Prevent/Correct Deformity ☐   Improve Ambulation ☐

Reduce Axial Load   ☐   Fracture Treatment ☐

Protect Joint   ☐   Other _____

ORTHOTIC RECOMMENDATION

LOWER LIMB		FLEX	EXT	ABD	ADD	ROTATION Int.	ROTATION Ext.	AXIAL LOAD
HKAO	Hip							
KAO	*Thigh*							
	Knee							
AFO	*Leg*							
	Ankle	(Dorsi)	(Plantar)					
	Subtalar					(Inver.)	(Ever.)	
FO Foot	Midtarsal							
	Met.-phal.							

REMARKS:

_____   _____

Signature   Date

KEY: Use the following symbols to indicate desired control of designated function:

F = FREE   — *Free* motion.

A = ASSIST   — Application of an external force for the purpose of increasing the range, velocity, or force of a motion.

R = RESIST   — Application of an external force for the purpose of decreasing the velocity or force of a motion.

S = STOP   — Inclusion of a static unit to deter an undesired motion in one direction.

v = Variable — A unit that can be adjusted without making a structural change.

H = HOLD   — Elimination of all motion in prescribed plane (verify position).

L = LOCK   — Device includes an optional lock.

Fig. 6.3 Functional descriptive classification: form for summary, treatment objectives and orthotic recommendation.

7

Ideal characteristics of orthoses

OBJECTIVES OF TREATMENT

Orthoses should be appropriate to achieve the medical objectives of treatment. This requires accurate, informed prescription and design both of mechanics and of structure.

LIGHTWEIGHT

Lightweight orthoses require choice of materials (compatible with reasonable cost) and design (see relationship between materials and structure—Appendix A).

RELIABILITY

Frequent breakage or failure of function is a grave disadvantage and this tends to increase with the complexity of orthosis. Primarily the need is for design and choice of materials, but help can also be rendered by rapid supply of modular parts and ease of local repair (this is an advantage of metal orthoses which can be repaired by non-specialists even in underdeveloped countries). Potential failure in this respect must dominate innovation. However good the orthosis it will not be acceptable if it is available one month in six or if it requires expert maintenance.

MANUFACTURING STANDARDS

The manufacturer should maintain high standards of material production and of quality control. This is a reason for central manufacturing of standard parts which can be incorporated in relatively locally-produced orthoses. This means that the numbers made make it economical to have accurate machinery in a production line with a high level of automation, good finishing and quality control. The various parts produced in this way, particularly in West Germany and the USA, are good examples of this. In the case of the ORLAU swivel walker, this is assembled to a near-finished state in an engineering workshop, and only the final modifications are made by the orthotist. This is possible because of accurate measurements facilitated by recording charts with provision of measuring jigs and the largely modular construction.

Control of materials is not always easy, as the producers of plastics dominated by the economics of the large-scale markets will modify these, on occasions, without an announcement. Recently polypropylene has been diluted with the cheaper polyethylene with loss of some valuable properties for the production of spring-like parts. By testing the products and insisting on certain standards of plastics, changes in materials can be detected and the orthosis design modified if necessary.

RAPID PROVISION AND REPLACEMENT

Again this points to a relatively large orthotic workshop maintaining a steady through-put. This necessitates a large population to be supplied, many of which will be a distance from the workshop. The fast transmission of information and orthoses to and from the workshop must be highly organized.

Modularity (i.e. the provision of standard parts of different shapes and sizes which can be partly or completely built into an orthosis) has been proposed as one solution with some limited success. It has the inherent difficulty that to be successful large stacks of components must be held, many of which may never be used. For the more complex orthoses it works, therefore, in special centres such as rehabilitation units for quadraplegics and treatment centres for scoliosis, and for paraplegics both congenital and traumatic. At the other end of the scale large numbers of 'off the shelf' products, belts, insoles and footdrop supports are being produced. These are successful if selection of the patient and modification on site is skilfully done.

ADJUSTABILITY

In the past a certain amount of material adjustment occurred with block leather devices under the influence of body heat and sweating. For this reason no patient was satisfied with a replacement, not realizing that a certain amount of usage had produced their previous comfortable state. Metal side bars can still be bent to some extent by the use of bending irons but plastic orthoses tend to maintain their original shape unless modified either by hammering in the case of high-density polyethylene (Ortholen), or with a heat gun for polypropylene.

COSMESIS

This must be both static and dynamic, including the elimination of noise on usage. The creaking of a long leg brace or the puff of a pneumatic valve can be equally disturbing. At the same time it must be realized that desirable as cosmesis is, it is not this that determines the acceptability of an orthosis but efficient function. There is no reason why they cannot be combined.

HYGIENE

The washability of plastics has been a bonus in their use.

SAFETY

This includes the avoidance of heat retention and allergic skin reaction. The latter may occur with metals, particularly zinc, and with some plastics. Fail-safe behaviour is supremely important. Single-sided long leg braces for stabilization have been recurrently advocated over a large number of years. Apart from their mechanical imperfections cases have been reported of breakage of such side bars, with fatal results from penetration of the femoral artery. To avoid dangerous breakage deliberate consideration must be given during design. In the hip guidance orthosis the hip joint construction is relatively brittle and can rarely break. To avoid any danger it is therefore backed with a ductile plate which will bend if this occurs but not break.

PATIENT ACCEPTABILITY

Patient acceptability includes a wide variety of factors:

1. Comfort on sitting as well as walking.
2. Ease of toilet functions.
3. Reasonable wear on clothes. Touch and close fastening is better than a number of straps and buckles, but it can play havoc with women's tights.
4. Ease of doff and don.
5. Low energy usage.
6. The 'X' factor in adoption of new devices which includes:
   (a) Novelty: particularly with research orthoses the early patients (often self-selecting and highly motivated) will be involved in the evolution of design, gradually becoming accustomed to the orthosis and gaining a semi-proprietorial interest in maintaining usage. This does not mean that it will be equally acceptable to the average newcomer.
   (b) The advice given to the patient. Some prescribers adopt a highly conservative attitude whilst others are willing to try every new device. Whatever standpoint is taken prescribers should make sure that they understand the device thoroughly and investigate the claims made for it before rejecting or accepting it.

PART III   REGIONAL AND NOSOLOGICAL CONSIDERATIONS

(To reduce repetition, these two classifications have been considered together)

8

Spinal orthoses

THE CERVICAL SPINE

The commonest conditions for which cervical orthoses are used are:

1. Cervical spondylosis (synonyms: degenerative disease, osteoarthritis), which rarely is associated with cervical disc prolapse.
2. Rheumatoid arthritis.
3. Trauma.
4. Infection, either acute or chronic.
5. Neoplasm—primary or secondary.
6. Osteoporosis.
7. Various neurological conditions causing profound muscle weakness and a consequent inability to maintain head posture.
8. Prevention of 'drop attacks' by limiting rotation and extension and therefore avoiding compression of vertebral arteries (probably already diseased).

Cervical spondylosis

It is widely recognized that considerable changes of this kind can be seen on X-rays without the patient having symptoms. The production of these is due to secondary inflammation.

Inflammation, it should be well understood, does not mean the same as infection. Whilst infection is a very common cause of inflammation it can occur as a result of strain. In consequence congestion and swelling (both in the capsule and within intervertebral joints) can occur, with associated pain deriving directly from the inflamed structures or secondarily from involvement of nerve root. A combination of inflammation and pressure (either swelling and/or prolapsed disc material) on nerve root or cord can produce pain in the limbs and/or neurological changes. Also, referred pain and tender areas can occur in the upper limbs and chest cage (Fig. 8.1). This is not due to involvement of nerve roots but comes from inflamed ligaments. It can, for example, mimic the symptoms of coronary thrombosis.

Objectives of treatment

The objectives of orthotic treatment are:

1.   To reduce inflammation and secondary spasm by resting in a chosen position.
2.   To relieve totally or partially compressive stress.
3.   To stabilize joints.
4.   To correct, prevent or support a fixed deformity.
5.   To limit joint range.
6.   To reduce heat loss.

Rest in a chosen position to reduce inflammation and secondary spasm

Because of the anatomy of the cervical spine (Fig. 8.2), there is a particularly close relationship between the intervertebral articulations which form part of the foramen and the emerging nerve roots. Loss of cartilage in these articulations with the formation of osteophytes results in considerable narrowing of the intervertebral foramen. If these joints then swell, either irritation or compression of the nerve can occur.

It is important to realize that these foraminae vary in shape with flexion and extension of the cervical spine and are open maximally in the slightly flexed position. Because of the usage of these collars in the past for such diseases as

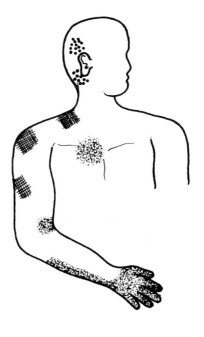
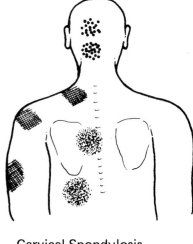

Cervical Spondylosis

 Upper

 Middle

 Lower

Fig. 8.1 Areas of pain and tenderness that can be referred from the cervical spine.

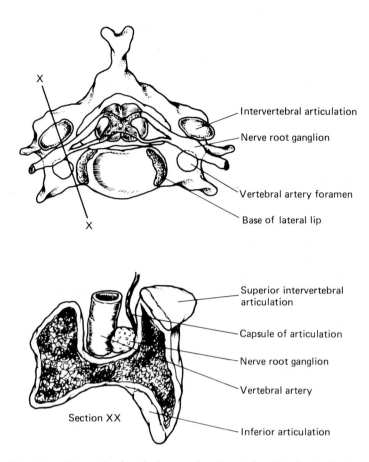

Intervertebral articulation

Nerve root ganglion

Vertebral artery foramen

Base of lateral lip

Superior intervertebral articulation

Capsule of articulation

Nerve root ganglion

Vertebral artery

Inferior articulation

Fig. 8.2 An oblique section from the foramen of a mid-cervical vertebra showing the close relationship between the capsule of the intervertebral articulation and the articulation itself.

tuberculosis of the spine for which extension of the neck was appropriate they may be routinely provided to maintain this position. In some circumstances this may aggravate both neck pain and brachial neuralgia.

In general patients are the best guide to the optimum position and their advice should be actively sought. There is no single brand that is suitable for all cases, and those fitting collars must have both the knowledge and facilities to modify these as required bearing in mind that the objective is to provide pain relief and not to replace one pain with another.

If in rheumatoid arthritis or infective conditions there is no danger of bony collapse the same criteria apply.

Total or partial relief of compressive stress

The forces producing this derive from:

1.   Gravitational—the weight of the head.
2.   Muscle spasm.

In spondylitis resting alone may relieve the spasm and to some extent a well-fitting rigid collar can provide some distraction between lower jaw and occipital above, and clavicular and thoracocervical junction below. Most importantly this function applies to those conditions in which there is a destructive element, trauma, infection (particularly the chronic infections such as tuberculosis), neoplasm, and to a lesser extent rheumatoid arthritis and osteoporosis. The greater the potential for collapse the more mechanically efficient and well fitting must be the orthosis. This may mean that it has to be brought down on to the chest or even to the pelvic rim with distraction being applied via a 'halo' attached directly by pins to the skull. Such orthoses have considerable advantages, as other forms of treatment, surgical and radiological for example, can be carried out without removal of the orthosis.

Stabilization of joints

Where there is deformity due to muscle weakness with full mobility in the cervical spine as in certain neurological disorders the chin comes to rest on the chest, impairing respiration, swallowing of food and vision. The best position in which to support the head will be such as to minimize the forces tending to cause recurrence, i.e. one of balance, and in this manner to reduce the demands on the orthosis, particularly at the interface. This position can be determined by the orthotist by simple trial whilst holding the head.

Correction, prevention or support of a fixed deformity

On occasions with the destructive conditions and with osteoporosis some improvement can be obtained in position by using a distraction type of orthosis. As in the correction of all fixed deformities, this requires the greatest continuous attention from the orthotist and prescriber in reducing the interface discomfort, increasing the correction when any gain is made and noting any signs of complication such as tingling or numbness. It also requires the highest level of cooperation and endurance from the patient. On occasions quite surprising improvement can be obtained but early recognition of the failure to achieve this is humane.

Limitation of joint range

In the cervical spine flexion–extension, lateral flexion and rotation are all limited to varying degrees by cervical orthoses. For any significant limitation of rotation a brace is mandatory.

Heat loss

The final function of cervical orthoses is to reduce heat loss.

Cervical orthoses, like lumbar, end up as, perhaps, one of the commonest forms of placebo.

Types of cervical orthoses

Cervical orthoses are rather arbitrarily divided into collars and braces without rigorous distinction (Fig. 8.3). In general a collar is limited to the neck and a brace will extend up the skull and/or downwards to the chest or pelvis. The degree of immobilization in even the most rigid and extensive braces is only moderate (Catachis, 1973; Johnson *et al.*, 1981; Zeleznik *et al.*, 1978) and by no means total, although the application of skeletal traction (halo traction) particularly with a well-moulded plastic pelvic girdle, approaches this most nearly.

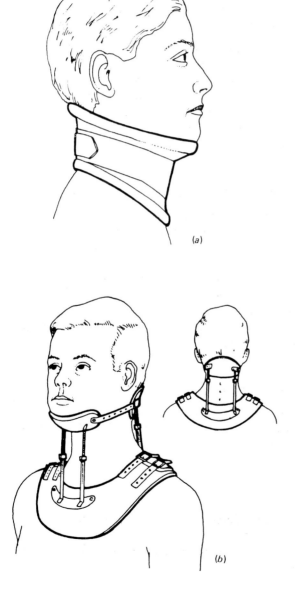

(a)

(b)

Fig. 8.3 (a) Collar. (b) Brace: distraction (four-poster) orthosis.

The commonly used mass-produced plastic foam collar is highly inefficient mechanically but has the advantage of immediate availability as does the slightly more efficient but relatively less comfortable collar made of padded rigid plastic, and inevitably a compromise has to be struck between the discomfort of the collar (which in some types can include high heat retention) and the symptoms of the condition itself. Failure to make substantial improvement with collars such as these should lead to discussion between prescriber, patient and orthotist regarding the more rigid types made of reinforced thermoplastic foams or block leather. One of the most important factors in providing these types of collars is getting the position correct from the very beginning. Although localized alterations can be made at a later stage, changes in the three-dimensional shape are virtually impossible. This applies both to secondary materials which are produced to a positive cast or materials which are applied to the patient.

Patients who are having a cast taken of their neck for the first time are inevitably nervous. If their medical condition allows the cast to be taken in a sitting position then this is always the easiest option for the orthotist. It is not always the case, especially after a fracture.

When the cast must be taken in two halves, posterior and anterior, it is essential that the patient relaxes the shoulder girdle which is usually elevated in nervous anticipation. If this is not done, when the patient stands the shoulders will drop and return to normal posture leaving the mandible and occiput totally unsupported. To stop this happening ask the patient to put his hands as far down the legs as possible whilst maintaining a supine position. Once the posterior shell has been completed, reinforce it and turn the patient with the cast in position. Then after greasing the edges complete the anterior shell. A Stryker rotating bed and several assistants are always a welcome sight when this difficult task is to be accomplished well. In rheumatoid arthritis, particularly, attention has to be paid not only to the problem of doff and don but of obtaining adequate closure to achieve maximum efficiency.

The distraction form of orthoses usually have four metallic pillars (four-poster) which are made so that one half slides out of the other and is controlled by a nut (Fig. 8.3(b)). This enables not only the degree of distraction to be modified but also the flexion/extension position of the neck.

A large number of patients can be fitted using a relatively small number of sizes, provided that at the upper end the mandibular and occipital pads (making purchase over as large an area as possible) are joined by adjustable straps; and that at the lower end as large as possible sternal and interscapular pads are similarly joined.

It is a useful device not only for treatment but also for safety protection, as for example when a suspected fracture of the cervical spine is being X-rayed, particularly if this is accompanied by any root or cord signs.

Clearly, when immobilization of the cervical spine is considered there are two problem areas: (1) the junction with the skull (the atlanto-occipital joint) and (2) the thoracocervical junction.

Any collar that is not circumferential about the neck clearly does not provide any significant immobilization here. Investigation of this problem has shown that:

1. The SOMI (sternomandibular occipital immobilizor; Johnson *et al.*, 1981) is the most efficient of all skeletal braces in limiting movement at upper point (Fig. 8.4). In the case of destructive and, therefore, potentially collapsing disease in this area, a block leather or plastic collar (Fig. 8.5) brought up high over the occiput and provided with a band which embraces the forehead is most efficient in all planes, whereas the SOMI is relatively inefficient in protecting against lateral flexion.
2. At the thoracocervical level a firm plastic foam of the type illustrated in Fig. 8.6 was found to be most efficient (Johnson *et al.*, 1981; Zeleznik *et al.*, 1978).

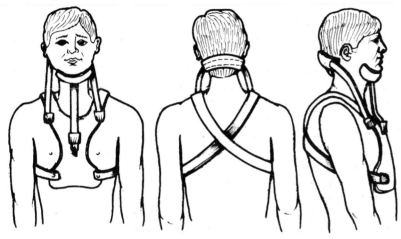

Fig. 8.4 SOMI brace— sternomandibular occipital immobilizer.

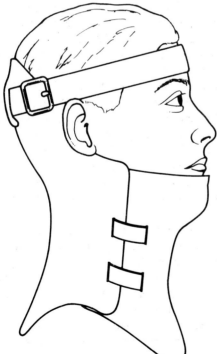

Fig. 8.5 Use of forehead band for high collapsing disease of upper cervical vertebrae.

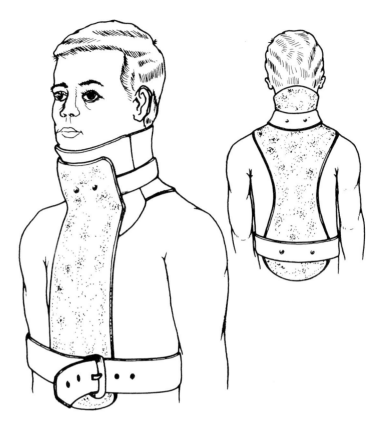

Fig. 8.6 Thoraco-cervical brace of rigid foam with fibreglass plates of similar rigid material (speckled).

THORACIC SPINE

The indications for orthoses here are as in the cervical region but the compressive forces of gravity are now considerably increased and cannot be so successfully resisted as those in the cervical region. Once again the important prognostic indicator for the successful use of orthoses is largely the difference between stabilization and support. The former occurs where the spine can be brought into the balanced position and the loading passes through the structures of the spine itself, or at any rate those that are intact.

To understand this some appreciation of the normal mechanics of the spine is necessary. In general the most efficient way of maintaining intrinsic stabilization of the human skeleton is to balance one bone upon another and then to use, under strict feedback control, appropriate muscular activity to restore this balance when it is lost for any reason. This seems unlikely when considering the multiple curves of the spine in the sagittal plane, but electromyography shows that in standing the normal spine requires no muscular activity from the erector spinae on the convex surface. This strongly suggests that equilibrium is being achieved, and this view is supported by the fact that if one considers each articulation in turn then balance only demands that the centre of gravity of the part of the body above that articulation should be over its axis. Experiments both with models and with frozen cadavers show that for chosen levels in the spine the relevant centre of mass will, in fact, be above the articulation (see Fig. 3.2, page 22).

Should flexion deformity of the spine occur due to progressive reduction, for any reason, of the height of the vertebral bodies and/or discs, then a continuing and increasing demand will be made on the appropriate muscles. Gradually this response will prove ineffective and progressive deformity accelerates as the mechanical advantage of gravity increases with the increasing deformity. No orthosis is then effective in resisting this, let alone correcting it. The solution, where appropriate, is to use gravity initially to correct the deformity, the patient being put into a recumbent position on a divided plaster bed.

Commonly in conditions such as ankylosing spondylitis a surprising degree of correction can be obtained quite rapidly in what appears to be a rigid spine. The initial hinge is chosen arbitrarily, but this is then modified to correspond with the point of correction when it becomes apparent.

However, if less than sufficient correction is obtained so that the standing

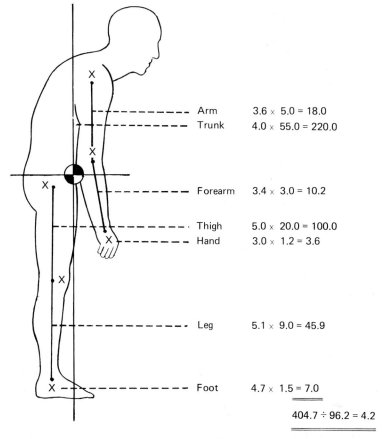

Arm	3.6 × 5.0 =	18.0
Trunk	4.0 × 55.0 =	220.0
Forearm	3.4 × 3.0 =	10.2
Thigh	5.0 × 20.0 =	100.0
Hand	3.0 × 1.2 =	3.6
Leg	5.1 × 9.0 =	45.9
Foot	4.7 × 1.5 =	7.0

404.7 ÷ 96.2 = 4.2

Fig. 8.7 Using the data provided by Dempster (1961) the centre of mass of the whole body or any portion can be calculated by summation of moments of individual segments about two ordinates at right angles. If the mobile articulation is known in any patient, the degree of correction necessary to produce stability can be determined.

patient requires to be supported then recurrence of the deformity is again very likely whatever orthosis is used. The safe position (in fact somewhat over centre) can be calculated using the free body technique combined with the data provided by Dempster (Fig. 8.7) and an appropriate orthosis then used.

In these circumstances a Jewett type of brace which relies on three-point fixation can be effective, which it is not as a support (Fig. 8.8). Support is somewhat better provided in those orthoses which endeavour to transmit this compressive force from axilla to the pelvic rim, for example the Fischer Jacket (Fig. 8.9). With modern materials and techniques very firm pelvic support can be achieved and tolerated as in the Milwaukee brace; but the axillary support, applied as it is to soft tissues and the mobile joint complex of the shoulder and scapular on the chest wall, is inefficient. Fortunately, with the advance of spinal surgery the need for such appliances in developed countries is now rare.

The factor of muscular activity within this type of brace as in the Milwaukee brace is an integral part of the concept of the orthoses. This should be particularly considered when dealing with patients suffering from progressive neuromuscular disease who can lose the ability to move away from discomfort. A child with muscular dystrophy can virtually hang himself within a Milwaukee brace as the spine collapses.

There have been a considerable number of variants in posterior spinal 'supports', but as has been indicated biomechanically these should be correctly used as stabilizers. Even with strong posterior components such as the Thomas–Jones back brace or the Taylor brace, they function mainly because increasing interface discomfort at the axilla reminds the patient that stability is being lost and induces active correction. In mechanical terms these are inherently highly inefficient as supporting devices, but act in cases of fixed defor-

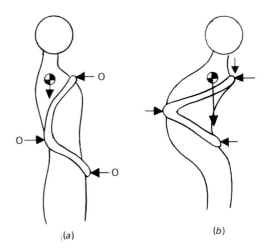

Fig. 8.8 Three-point fixation in a Jewett brace. (a) The brace is eminently satisfactory when used as a stabilizer. (b) The brace is unsatisfactory when used as a support. In (a) The centre of mass is over the point of articulation and there is no collapsing moment; in (b) there is a turning moment which is not resisted to any significant extent by the three-point fixation. The sternum and pelvis tend to come closer together and need traction to prevent this.

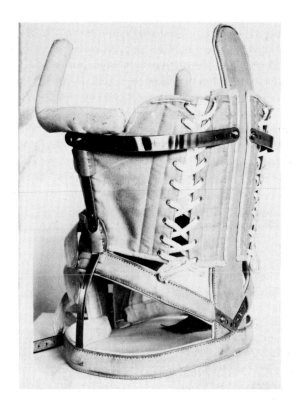

Fig. 8.9 Fischer jacket designed in principle to provide support or distraction, but there can be interface problems at the upper end.

mity, as in a quiescent tuberculosis of the spine, by reducing the flexion movement in the affected area. They become, therefore, rest devices; but they cannot be expected to prevent collapse in active disease.

THE LUMBAR SPINE

The medical conditions for which lumbar orthoses are used are again similar to other areas of the spine, but are dominated statistically by back ache and sciatica, the orthoses for which make up 25 per cent of the total national orthotic budget and account for 33 per cent of the total number of orthoses supplied. Empirically, those with back ache often feel an instinctive need for something firm wrapped round this area, and this form of relief has probably been supplied for centuries. There are now over 50 types of lumbar and sacro-iliac supports, many with eponymous names, so even at this time it is not possible to make a dogmatic statement regarding the precise function or effectiveness of these. Many of them often bear now only a modest resemblance to the original description of the support. For many, design is simply traditional and no precise designs are available. In consequence regional variations may develop so that a Goldthwait orthosis (note the absence of the final 'e' so often added to the name) can look and function in many different ways depending on which part of the country it is manufactured and this reflects the considerable confusion that surrounds this type of orthosis.

Again, they are rather arbitrarily divided into braces which are mainly solid in construction, and corsets which are mainly made of varying mixtures of fabrics. Amongst the braces are the Goldthwait, the Knight Chair back, the McKee and Jordan types, to which have been added recently a variety made of plastic. To the corset are added varying degrees of posterior rigid framework or plates with the intention of applying local pressure and restricting movements, plus other steels or bones to the sides. These are often added to resist the tendency for soft material to concertina, particularly in patients who have a reasonable waist, when tightened, due to the normal resolution of forces.

In general, concepts of functions fall into the following groups:

1. To rest joints and associated soft structures.
2. Relief of compressive stress.
3. Pressure on local areas of tenderness.
4. Heat retention.
5. Placebo effect.

Rest of joints and associated soft structures

The technical problems of trying to immobilize this area derive from:

1. The anatomical situation, i.e. the number of joints sited close together and covered by muscle masses, making the application of restraining force to a particular area extremely difficult.
2. The long leverage of the body and the weight of the trunk which makes the moments to be resisted considerable.

Furthermore, the shape of the back varies from standing to bending. This implies the need for an articulated corset which restrains movement in a small area of the lower spine, but attempts to provide this have met with no real success.

Three possible translations of motion exist: (a) sagittal; (b) coronal; (c) horizontal rotation of the spine compared with the pelvis around a vertical axis.

Efficiency of immobilization has been investigated (Ahlgren and Hansen, 1978; Deane and Grew, 1978; Norton and Brown, 1957; Rubin *et al.*, 1972). Only about 15 per cent of horizontal movement is reduced by a corset, compared with some 70 per cent in plaster jackets. These are generally more effective in reducing all translations than are corsets but long supports that have a good purchase around the shoulder actually increase the range of movement in the lumbosacral region. Such investigations are of limited value, not only because the conditions under which they are done tend to be very artificial, but clinical experience shows that the position of immobilization can be as important as the degree. For example, patients put into a plaster corset, particularly under some traction, can occasionally have a substantial increase in pain rather than relief. This is particularly the case where the patient has an antalgic posture, i.e. a position that minimizes nerve root pressure or irritation. It is this, and not muscle spasm which produces the so-called sciatic scoliosis of the lumbosacral disc protrusion or the reversed lordosis of the L4–5 disc. Straightening and limiting the spinal position will obliterate this optimum position with adverse results. Once again the patient can provide information in regard to the position of immobilization.

It has been postulated by Raney and others that flexion of the lumbar spine is helpful and he has designed a support to provide this which also has a scaphoid indentation of the abdomen to enhance intra-abdominal pressure. Another variant of this is the Boston Overlap brace. It is made in thinner materials than the Boston Scoliosis brace, has a front opening with overlap and comes in modules. The usefulness of this position is hotly debated but again the best guide to its usage is the comfort of the patient in this position. Protagonists claim, however, that this cannot be determined immediately and that the patient must expect some initial discomfort from the skin-tight orthosis.

It also emerged that the effectiveness of support seemed to be related more to the discomfort produced on movement than the magnitude of force developed between the orthosis and the back and it appears that inhibition rather than mechanical resistance should be one essential feature. As one would expect, extrinsic factors can also modify the situation and in particular tightness of the hamstrings. If this is present an increased strain on the lumbar spine will be produced on forward flexion, and the necessary instruction for all belt users in correct lifting and bending techniques needs to be emphasized.

Whilst some discomfort may be inhibitory and acceptable a more severe degree will lead to the abandonment of the orthosis, whilst careful attention to this point can maintain the patient even in heavy work such as farm labouring. Common causes of abandonment due to discomfort are:

1. Irritation of and pressure on the groin in the sitting position. Careful tailoring of the lower edge is needed, high enough to avoid this problem but low enough to prevent the protrusion and subsequent compression of the abdominal fat below the belt.

2. The tendency of the support to ride up resulting in poor fit and the appreciation by the patient that the comforting compression is not in the correct place. The problem is most easily dealt with in women by the use of stockings and suspenders but in men the classic solution was the use of groin straps. These are almost universally abandoned because of discomfort. A useful solution is a 'Tubigrip skirt'. An appropriate diameter Tubigrip is put on initially from the nipple line to just below the knee and the belt then assumed. The lower portion of the Tubigrip is then turned upwards to form a double thickness which extends over the belt but leaves a 'skirt' which embraces the buttocks with a slight redundancy at the lower edge. This forms a comfortable thickening below the buttock folds and holds both Tubigrip and belt down into position. Because of its elasticity the front can be higher than the back to provide comfort in the groin.

It is commonly assumed that the wearing of these belts causes muscular atrophy. Investigation into this subject (Waters and Morris, 1970) has shown that for both a corset and a brace the back muscles are not affected while walking at a normal pace, and there is some increased activity at a fast pace when wearing a brace. This is thought to be due to the reduction of horizontal pelvic translation. On the other hand, the abdominal musculature under all circumstances is either not affected or decreased.

This suggests that the effect of lumbosacral supports on back musculature has been exaggerated but that abdominal exercises are probably a necessary adjunct to the belt support, particularly as these can be achieved painlessly, whereas even isometric back exercises commonly cause a recrudescence of pain.

In general advice given about the wearing of belts seems to be often rather arbitrary and theoretically poorly based. It would seem logical that if one wished to rest an inflamed area, initial immobilization should be continuous. Clinical experience shows that good results are obtained if a very firm belt or brace is worn initially during the waking hours until the pain has largely disappeared. In these circumstances a lighter belt can then be supplied and as this gradually wears, becoming less efficient, it allows the safe transfer of support to the muscle. Important advice is that the belt should not be thrown away when symptoms have subsided, so that in the event of recurrence it can be used immediately and will then often abort a prolonged attack which may occur if time and money is wasted in the process of obtaining a new one.

Because of the effectiveness in some circumstances of narrow belts which clearly have little mechanical effect on the lumbosacral level, other theories of functions have been suggested:

1. That narrow belts can impose a beneficial posture. It is often assumed that 'beneficial' in these terms means as near to normal as possible, but this has been considerably debated and there is a school of thought that advocates elimination of the lumbar lordosis (Raney, 1969). Certainly this has been beneficial in some cases but not all. A recent addition to the family of lumbosacral braces is the Boston Overlap which imposes this posture, and is to some extent adjustable.
2. That these might diminish the posterior subluxation of the facet joints if correctly placed, as in Fig. 8.10(a).
3. That they could limit the wedge-like action of the sacrum in relationship to sacro-iliac joints under the effect of body weight. Whilst the diagnosis 'sacro-iliac strain' has been eclipsed by the problems of the lumbosacral complex, the success of such belts and the use of a narrow belt by professional weightlifters tends to support the fact that it remains a genuine clinical entity (Fig. 8.10(b)).

The essential problem in the prescription of orthoses for low-back pain remains the difficulty in providing a precise diagnosis and then prescribing treat-

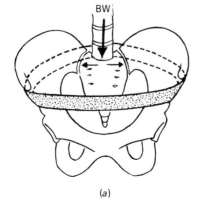
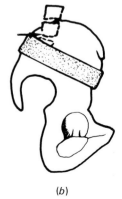

Fig. 8.10 (a) Theoretical function of a narrow band incorporated into a lumbosacral corset to oppose the wedge separation of the sacro-iliac joints under body weight (BW). (b) This opposes the posterior subluxation of the lumbosacral articulations.

(a)

(b)

ment that matches the need. To some extent, therefore, treatment is of necessity empirical and this has been embodied in a form of belt which is modular in type and which can be modified according to the patient's response. A narrow sacro-iliac type of belt is provided in the first instance, but this can be extended upwards to provide increasing coverage and potential support by an appropriate system of touch-and-close attachments (Velcro, straps, bands, pads and steels). Regrettably, this excellent concept does not seem to have attracted the attention of the prescriber that it deserves, and production at this time seems to have been discontinued.

Relief of compressive stresses

An important factor recognized in the last 20 years has been the relationship of abdominal pressure with the mechanical stresses on the lumbar spine (Davies, 1956, 1959; Davies and Troup, 1964). Experiments have shown that in forward bending, unless a rise in intra-abdominal pressure occurs, forces beyond 'safe loading' can be imposed on the lower lumbar spine. Firm compression of the abdominal wall can enhance intra-abdominal pressure and attention has been directed to this area of the belt.

It has been demonstrated that an inflatable pad placed within the front of the corset can considerably raise this pressure thus lowering the static loading of the spine accompanied by a marked reduction in abdominal muscular activity, indicating that at this time function of the muscles was taken over by the corset. However, during activity there was little, if any, difference in the maximum pressure on the abdomen with and without the corset. It seems therefore that such an inflatable device is useful for standing pain but abdominal exercises are indicated for pain of movement. It is also obvious that the efficiency of any belt in this respect is reduced if the patient has either a large diaphragmatic hernia or gross pelvic prolapse and indeed that in these circumstances only a skeletal type of brace which cannot aggravate these conditions should be used.

Relief of pressure

It is a matter of empirical experience that some help is obtained from pressure on local areas of tenderness, although not necessarily all. Experimentation will indicate the need for an appropriate pad in this position in the placement of which the patient's guidance is invaluable.

Heat rentention

In the elderly (Dixon *et al.*, 1972) the beneficial effect of heat retention has been demonstrated and an extra appropriate heat-retaining layer may well be useful. In other instances, however, with patients working in warm environments or abroad, this retention may be a considerable problem and can be dealt with to some extent by the use of skeletal braces or open-wove material in corsets, although the latter has to be balanced against the diminution in other functions.

Placebo effect

The placebo effect related to neurotics and litigants is well recognized statistically but difficult to identify individually.

Overall, therefore, whilst the inability of the prescriber in many circumstances to make a precise diagnosis has to be recognized and the effects of orthoses are multiple and variable in functional terms, this does not absolve either the prescriber or orthotist from providing that orthosis most likely to be effectual and to modify the prescription in the light of follow-up. Failure to do this has led to these orthoses being under-valued, although with proper control they can be highly beneficial and carry a lower morbidity and even mortality than some other forms of treatment.

SCOLIOSIS

This is dealt with as a separate subject because of the potential effects on all levels of the spine and because there have been more variations in design and concepts, in unwarranted optimism and in pessimism than in any other form of orthosis. In the main this derives from two factors:

1. The very considerable mechanical problems:
    (a) The deforming segments are multiple and small so that it is difficult to concentrate the corrective force at the primary site of deformity.
    (b) The segments are a relatively long distance from the point of application of the correcting force. Where this is applied through another segment, e.g. the ribs, these segments are themselves likely to deform before correcting the deformity, particularly if the force is not applied along their long axis.
    (c) The rotational nature of the deformity requiring correcting forces in all planes.
2. The essential nature of the condition, arising during growth and consequent upon muscle imbalance of a paralytic condition or the possible localized failure of tissue development in the idiopathic form. Both of these are then likely to produce forces that are more efficient in deformation than the orthosis can be in correction.

Fortunately, these orthoses have been submitted to a greater degree of critical assessment and scientific development than almost any others. An important baseline of the prognostic pattern of scoliosis had been established (Ponseti and Friedman, 1950; James, 1959, 1960) and this means that the effect of an orthosis can be measured against the natural history. In infantile scoliosis, for example, it is known that in most cases (and there are now ways of identifying the others) the natural history is that of complete cure; consequently, orthotic treatment has been abandoned.

Relatively early in the history of plaster-of-Paris jackets supplied for this condition (Abbott, 1911), the contribution of internally generated forces reacting against the orthosis was appreciated. This is a fundamental part of modern treatment, going some way to match the problem in (2) above. It is for this reason that whilst the Milwaukee brace and its direct descendant the Boston brace will use external pads distributed on mechanical principles, integrated exercise therapy is regarded as essential. It is now believed that the internally generated forces can be regarded as the most important, if not the only corrective mechanism. That this is likely to be the case is evident from consideration of the system's total energy.

Use of a mechanical three-point system applied to a 'fixed' deformity implies that if it is to be successful, there will be some yielding in this deformity, and therefore energy derived from external forces at the time of application of the orthosis will be stored in this yielding area. It will be released if and when the deformity diminishes or if the orthosis is taken off. Once this has happened re-application of the unmodified orthosis can produce no further result. Modification may be obtained by straps which can be tightened or by introducing larger pads within an unchanging outer mould, a technique first described in 1911 (Abbott). It follows that a mechanical jacket or brace which is entirely comfortable for a substantial proportion of its life can in fact exert no mechanical effect. (In the former method, it would seem better that the design would allow modification to be done in small optimum steps rather than by the arbitrarily chosen intervals dictated by holes in the straps. Indeed Stagnera, a French orthopaedic surgeon, uses a ratchet device in these circumstances.)

It has been suggested that the built-in lumbar flexion of the Boston brace brings the transverse processes of the curved lumbar vertebrae to a point where they can be reached by pads to exert correctional forces. This has a secondary requirement, namely that the brace should extend as far as it is necessary above and below to maintain this flexed posture.

Another aspect of orthotic design (Hall and Miller, 1963) is illustrated in relation to interface and subcutaneous pressures with these devices, where emphasis is placed on the waisting of the pelvic component to position adequate tissue between the shelf so produced and the iliac crest.

Use of plastic pelvic modules has been exploited in both cases, producing rapid supply and consistency of design. Importantly, protagonists of the Boston brace claim that these modules can correct lumbar, thoracolumbar and lower thoracic curves without the metal superstructure which can be a source of embarrassment to patients when wearing the Milwaukee. As in all these situations, a strict protocol must be observed and this is made possible by the provision of very adequate detailed data (Hall and Miller, 1963; Watts *et al.*, 1977, 1979) provided by the initiator to indicate principles, indications and contra-indications, follow-up, instructions to the patients, and details of physical therapy combined with photographic and radiographic recording. No complex orthosis is complete without such instruction and the production of this is not only useful to the prescriber but equally to the innovator. The writing of such a document highlights what is proved and what is hypothesis, and what yet remains to be done in the clinical and research field.

A most useful instruction for the Boston brace is concerned with the production of a 'blueprint' for the orthotist. The whole spine and ribs are X-rayed in the standing position with a radio-opaque plumb-line. On this film a line is drawn vertically through the spinous process of S1 and a transverse line across the superior edge of each iliac crest. The curves are measured by the Cobb method (Fig. 8.11) as is wedging and deviation of each vertebra from the vertical. Particularly important is the identification of the 'null point' of the curve, at

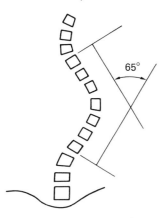

Fig. 8.11 The Cobb angle is used to measure the degree of curve. The highest body of the curve is that in which a line drawn across the superior surfaces tilts into the concavity, and the lowest that in which a line drawn through the inferior surface tilts similarly.

which deviation of the vertebrae hinges from right to left or vice versa. Axial rotation is also determined. From this 'blueprint' both placement of pads and the 'trim line' are determined. If this procedure were to be undertaken for every case of scoliosis fitted with an orthosis, considerable enlargement of the understanding of both prescriber and orthotist would occur with consequent improvement in treatment standards. The overall lesson is that no orthosis is automatic in its function and that each case demands individual consideration and understanding of the orthotic principles, whatever the complexity of the splint.

In the treatment of scoliosis, orthotic–surgical integration is extremely important. This problem is one, therefore, where a team approach is highly developed. Blount (Blount and Moe, 1973) has provided guidance regarding the age and degree of curve likely to need orthotic correction, and this method should be applied to those in other zones of the graph (Fig. 8.12).

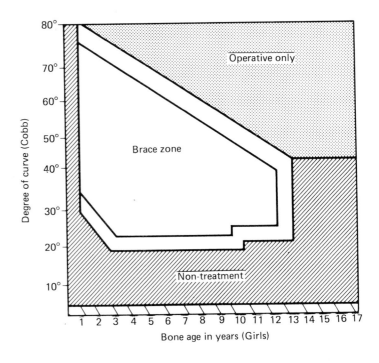

Fig. 8.12 Brace zone after Blount.

9

Hand and wrist orthoses

Conditions for which these are commonly used are:

1. Trauma—the supply has increased lately due to application of functional fracture bracing (cast-brace) principles (see page 166).
2. Rheumatoid arthritis.
3. Neurological conditions, including flaccid and spastic paralysis with and without sensory involvement.
4. Rarely in infective conditions.

The hand presents particular difficulties in orthotic treatment:

1. There is a vicious tendency to swell and stiffen. Both are minimized by movement and the avoidance of constriction.
2. The complex function requires a detailed knowledge of functional anatomy of:
   (a) Various grips in relationship to position of fixation, e.g. power (cylindrical (Fig. 9.1), spherical, hook grasp), precision (palmar (Fig. 9.2), tip, lateral pinch). It is particularly important to appreciate that as the fingers close they converge and alter in relative lengths (Fig. 9.2(b)).
   (b) Sensory loss related to nerve injury, because unnecessary coverage of residual normal sensory areas inhibits motor functions (Fig. 9.3); and because pressure in areas of sensory loss can cause thinning of subcutaneous tissue and/or ulceration. The shear-relieving functions of subcutaneous tissue (discussed in Chapter 13 on the foot) can be just as important, although the stresses are generally less.
3. Position of fingers related to ligamentous laxity—all joints should be immobilized with ligaments in tense position. If this is done with ligaments relaxed they will shorten and movement will be limited in future.
4. Joint axes in relationship to surface anatomy, e.g. axes of metacarpophalangeal joints compared with palmar creases (Fig. 9.4).
5. Transverse arches of hand, and need to maintain these (Fig. 9.5).

From the point of view of biomechanical classification, hand and wrist orthoses may be divided into those that:

1. Rest a joint or fracture in a chosen position.
2. Correct a 'fixed' deformity.
3. Exercise muscles and joints by dynamic splints.

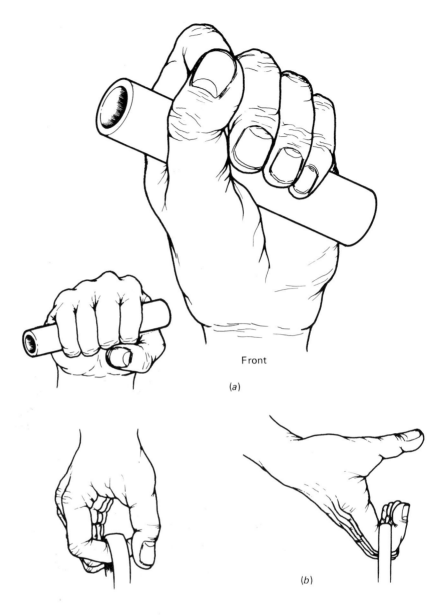

Front

(a)

(b)

Fig. 9.1 (a) Cylindrical power grip. Note the convergence of the fingers as in Fig. 9.2. (b) Hook grasp. This can be an important residual function in the very paralysed hand, either as a result of contracture or surgery.

4. Control joint range.
5. Transmit forces.
6. Provide coverage.

RESTING A JOINT OR FRACTURE IN A CHOSEN POSITION

In resting a fracture there are two considerations:

1. Prevention of re-deformity after reduction.
2. The minimization of stiffness occurring in neighbouring joints, and particularly in the digits during the necessary period of immobilization.

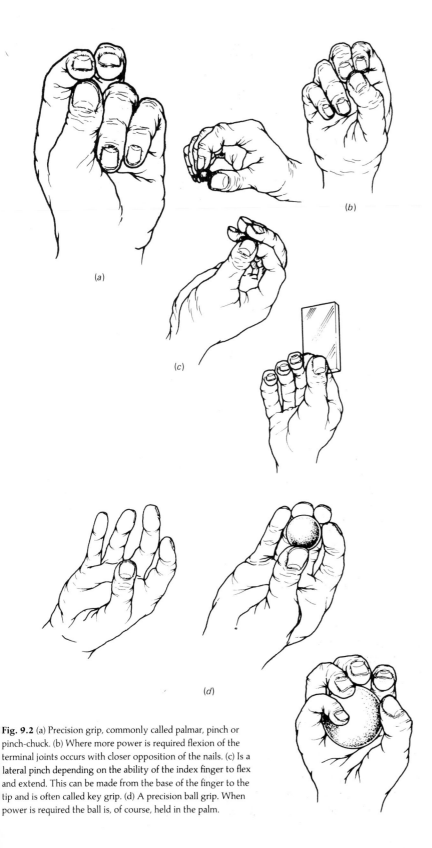

Fig. 9.2 (a) Precision grip, commonly called palmar, pinch or pinch-chuck. (b) Where more power is required flexion of the terminal joints occurs with closer opposition of the nails. (c) Is a lateral pinch depending on the ability of the index finger to flex and extend. This can be made from the base of the finger to the tip and is often called key grip. (d) A precision ball grip. When power is required the ball is, of course, held in the palm.

There may be some mutual antagonism in these aims which has accounted for the popularity of primary internal fixation for many of these fractures.

Where a fracture is broken into several pieces, i.e. comminuted (as in the 'Colles'' fracture posteriorly, Fig. 9.6), some collapse of the fracture site will occur under the influence of muscle activity even though initial alignment is achieved, because of the lack of mechanical stabilization provided by two intact fragments.

To try to prevent this attempts were made in the past to hold the distal fragment in position by using the tensioned posterior capsule of the wrist joint. This requires the hand be placed in full flexion and this so defunctions the fingers that the patient cannot exercise adequately, and stiffness may develop which is more disabling than some slight re-deformation of the fracture.

The optimum position is with the carpus in line with the radius, as this aligns the tendons of the flexors and extensors with the distal fragment, and reduces the potential deformity mechanism from these substantially to nil.

No joints should be immobilized unless this is necessary. If this applies to the metacarpo-phalangeal joints it is not always understood that the plaster or orthosis must not go beyond the proximal crease of the palm. In finger frac-

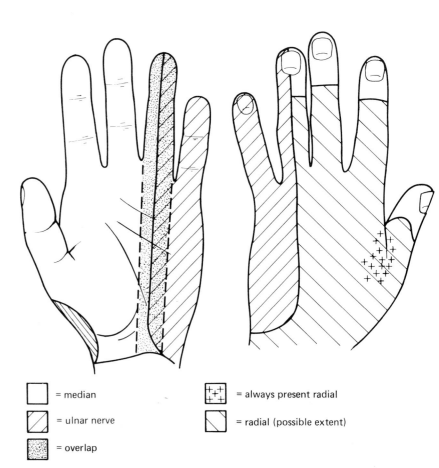

Fig. 9.3 Nerve distribution of the hand. Loss of the median nerve affects a large area of the front of the hand, particularly concerned with the precision grip and is functionally very inhibiting, whereas the ulnar loss is not so important.

☐ = median

◩ = ulnar nerve

▨ = overlap

⊞ = always present radial

◹ = radial (possible extent)

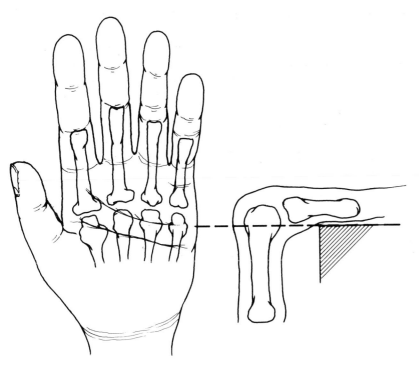

Fig. 9.4 The relationship of the metacarpal heads to the palmar creases. If full flexion of the metacarpo-phalangeal joints is to be allowed it will be seen that the critical level of the plaster is over the metacarpal necks, not the heads. The situation is similar in regard to the interphalangeal joints.

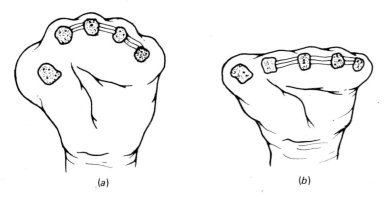

Fig. 9.5 (a) The normal curved position of the metacarpal heads. If as in (b) this is flattened, the metacarpo-phalangeal joints tend to stiffen and if flexion is achieved the normal convergence of the fingers is lost. If the thumb is also placed in line, the so-called simian (monkey) position, there will be marked dysfunction of the whole hand.

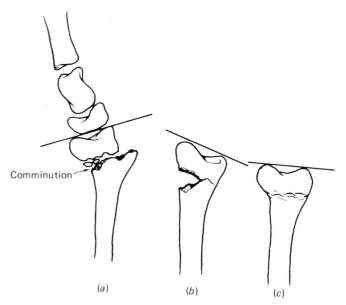

Fig. 9.6 (a) Colles' fracture of the wrist, lateral view with typical deformity, a displacement and tilting backwards of the distal fragment of the radius. (b) Anatomical reduction. (c) Common type of subsequent collapse as the comminuted (broken-up) fracture posteriorly does not provide inherent stability and the best orthosis may not be able to resist this deformity consequent upon muscle action.

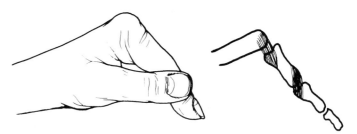

Fig. 9.7 The 'Edinburgh position'. In this position because of the relationship of the ligaments to the axis of the joints, they are at their tightest and cannot, therefore, shorten during the period of immobilization.

tures because of the complexity of normal and abnormal intrinsic muscle activity in relation to the fracture site the optimum results are achieved by the 'Edinburgh position' (Fig. 9.7). The metacarpo-phalangeal joint is the key joint of a finger and when splinted should be in flexion. This is because the ligaments which run each side of the joint obliquely are tightest in this position. If these joints are left extended or even worse hyperextended, the initially slack ligaments will now shorten in this position and flexion becomes either extremely difficult or impossible, with a gross reduction in the function of the hand. In the treatment of all disease prevention is better than cure, and in the hand this is particularly important as often the deformities once acquired cannot be cured.

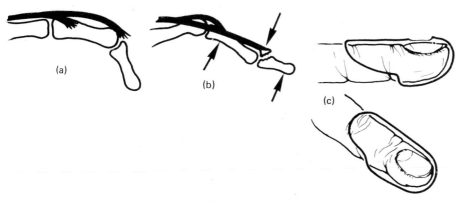

Fig. 9.8 Mallet finger; tearing of the tendon from the bone as in (a), or a small fragment of the bone as in (b). Here it can be seen that the three-point fixation necessary for the correction of the deformity tends to press over the vulnerable area of the lesion. (c) Polypropylene orthosis, proximal end is secured by circumferential strapping.

Specific examples

Specific examples of trauma orthoses are:

1. For mallet finger.
2. For middle slip (boutonnière) tear.
3. For lateral instability.
4. For rheumatoid arthritis.

Mallet finger

Here three-point fixation is used to try to oppose either the extensor tendon torn from the base of the distal phalanx posterior or the tendon plus a small fragment of bone. To attempt this (and it is unrealistic to believe that if any separation has occurred this gap will be closed), the distal joint is hyperextended and the proximal may be flexed to allow relaxation of the extensor tendon which occurs when the lateral slips of extensor hood of the proximal interphalangeal joint move to the sides of the joint in this position (Fig. 9.8). If a short anterior splint is used care must be taken to see that it allows full flexion of the proximal interphalangeal joint. Otherwise, when this is done the splint will be pushed distally becoming ineffective, and any strapping holding it in position tightened with adverse pressure results. What one is in fact achieving is:

1. Resting the area so that it heals as promptly as possible with least pain.
2. Preventing further separation of torn-out extensor mechanism with the development of a right-angle deformity. This is a significant disability, whereas a slight loss of extension is none.
3. Protecting against knocks.

A practical problem is that one point of the three-point fixation presses directly on the damaged area which in any case is thinly covered with skin and soft tissue, so that too great a pressure here may produce skin breakdown.

The common orthoses now used are standard rigid plastic 'finger stalls' (Fig. 9.8(c)).

Middle slip or boutonnière (button-hole) tear

This occurs in the middle slip of the extensor hood of the proximal interphalangeal joint (Fig. 9.9). It is produced by traumatic laceration or spontaneous rupture in rheumatoid arthritis. As in the mallet finger an attempt is made to get the torn ends in apposition by positioning the finger. This is done by the use of three-point fixation, in this case with the finger straight using a wire or plastic splint.

Lateral instability

Lateral instability can be dealt with by a similar skeletal device appropriately positioned.

Rheumatoid arthritis

In rheumatoid arthritis swan neck deformity occurs (Fig. 9.10), the reverse of that in the middle slip tear. It can look horrifying, but two types exist. One is actively correctable by the patient and for this no orthosis is indicated nor indeed will it be tolerated by the patient. The one that is correctable, but only passively, is a considerable handicap and an orthosis that maintains the proximal phalangeal joint in some flexion substantially improves hand function.

Maintenance of function

The particular function of the hand demands an orthotic criterion not so

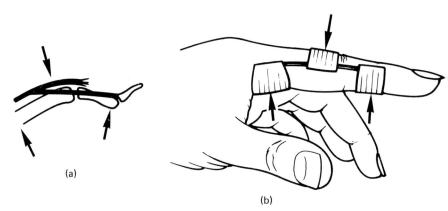

(a)

(b)

Fig. 9.9 Middle slip or boutonnière tear. It produces the characteristic deformity (a) and is treated with a rigid three point fixation (b). This has the advantage that the posterior point is not over the site of the lesion.

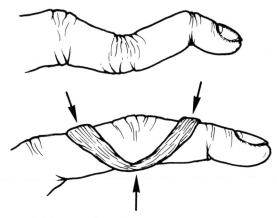

Fig. 9.10 'Swan neck' deformity with simple low-temperature mouldable plastic orthosis which must be moulded individually for each patient.

important elsewhere—namely to maintain a functional position. For example, if there is a loss of abduction of the thumb due to median nerve palsy or a direct injury to the thenar muscles, the thumb will tend to lie in line with the hand (the simian or monkey position, Fig. 9.11), and the pinch grip between index finger and thumb tip is not possible. An orthosis (an opponens type) that holds the thumb abducted will improve the function of the index finger. In the median nerve lesion there will also be weakness of flexion of the terminal joint of the index finger and this will be helped by a slip-on tubular orthosis to hold the joint in slight flexion. In this lesion there is considerable inhibition of function due to the sensory loss. No orthosis can improve this.

Another area to which attention must be paid is the transverse arch of the metacarpals which is normally concave anteriorly; if this flattens, or worse, is reversed the normal convergence of the fingers is lost as is the deepening of the palm, both of which enable normal 'ball' grasp to be made. Here as in other situations, maintenance of the curve with mobility is ideal.

CORRECTION OF A 'FIXED' DEFORMITY

Clearly the word fixed must be qualified. Absolute fixation permits no correction orthotically and success depends on stretching the scar tissue (particularly when this is immature) and contracted ligaments (as indicated, better prevented). It depends on constant progressive application of force, limited by skin pressure tolerance, to the contracted area. This can be done either actively or passively.

Active correction

The energy for active correction can be provided either directly by the patient's own muscles or by stored energy in some elastic or spring device. When using the patient's own muscles, the problem is to localize the appli-

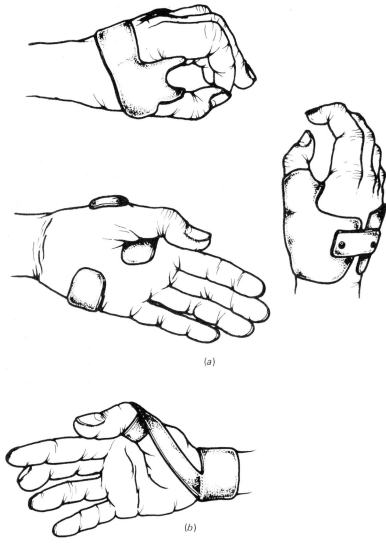

Fig. 9.11 Opponens orthoses (a) to fix the thumb in the best functional position. (b) Is a lively orthosis, the thumb being held by an elastic band. It enables the non-paralysed muscles around the thumb to be exercised, but when a pinch grip is attempted it relies on the limitation of the basal joint of the thumb to react against the force applied to the tip. Functionally it is therefore inefficient but may prevent stiffness developing in the simian position during recovery.

cation of these to the affected joints. Where a number of joints are close together, as in the fingers, muscular activity will move mobile joints to their full range and have no effect on the contracted joints. If, for example, the proximal interphalangeal joints of the fingers did not flex fully, only by limiting the movement in the metacarpo-phalangeal joints, so that the force of the flexor muscles may be applied to the contracted joints, can (often quite rapid) improvement occur (see Fig. 2.5, page 14).

If stored energy is to be used in a similar situation, the device shown in Fig. 5.19 (page 54) would be characteristic. The energy is loaded during the application of the splint and care should be taken to see that the strength of the elastic or spring is just less than that of the muscles opposing the stretching. This has two advantages:

1. By using these muscles the patient can intermittently relieve the stress on the scar tissue should this become too painful (although it must be said that it is better to supply a slow continuous stretching than an intermittent fierce one which is more likely to damage the immature scar and produce reactive thickening and further contracture).
2. Any extensor movement present in the finger is maintained whilst the flexion is being improved.

Passive stretching

Passive stretching is produced by a rigid device of a shape designed to stretch tight tissues slightly when applied. The energy for this comes from the patient or person initially applying the orthosis. As stretching occurs so that it can be put on easily, it is obviously ineffective and needs constant modification. In the case of a plaster-of-Paris cast this may involve repeated wedging, or a turnbuckle may be incorporated into an orthosis, as for stretching a flexion deformity of wrist or elbow (Fig. 9.12).

The general rule is to make sure that all stretching force is applied to the contracted joint or joints, and to avoid distortion of the others.

EXERCISE OF MUSCLE AND JOINTS

The orthosis may be required to exercise muscle and joints by means of dynamic or lively splints designed to replace paralysed musculature so that all joints can be put through a full range of movement and thus avoid deformity and at the same time exercise and maintain the intact musculature. It was once thought that by preventing paralysed muscles from becoming 'over stretched' functional recovery could be hastened as the muscle was then in better condition to re-function once reinnervation occurred. There is, in fact, very little evidence to support this; and provided that the joints are maintained in full mobility by one way or another, splintage is not absolutely necessary, particularly if it involves multiple and sometimes dangerous wire structures.

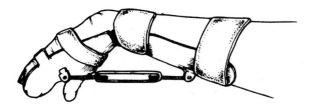

Fig. 9.12 A turnbuckle for passive stretching of a wrist flexion contracture.

Examples of splints used in this way are:

1. Wrist and metacarpo-phalangeal joint assistors in radial nerve palsy (Fig. 9.13).
2. An opponens splint for median nerve palsy (see Fig. 9.11(a)).
3. A spring-loaded 'knuckleduster' for ulnar nerve palsy (Fig. 9.14).

CONTROL OF JOINT RANGE

Post-operatively in rheumatoid arthritis after the insertion of Silastic joints the requirement is to maintain the normal aligned range of movement but to prevent, in the early stages, abnormal movements such as recurrence of ulnar deviation at the metacarpo-phalangeal joints.

TRANSMISSION OF FORCES

The classic example of this is the wrist-driven flexor hinge orthosis (see Fig. 5.28, page 62).

COVERAGE

Coverage is largely protective and very much overlaps the resting splints. It is particularly useful in bed, when the rheumatoid or post-traumatic hand may be aggravated by uncontrolled patient movement.

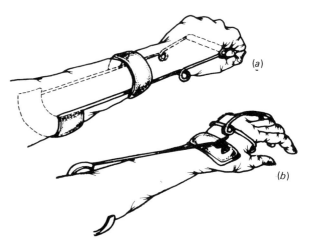

Fig. 9.13 (a) A wrist assistor for a partial radial nerve palsy affecting wrist extensors only. (b) In a complete palsy the matacarpo-phalangeal joints will also drop and extensions will be necessary for the fingers and thumb. In these circumstances great care must be taken not to hyperextend these joints.

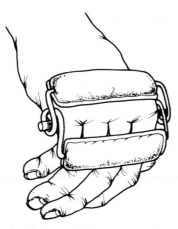

Fig. 9.14 A spring-loaded 'knuckleduster' for ulnar nerve palsy. It opposes the hyperextension of the ulnar two metacarpo-phalangeal joints which occurs with this. It prevents stiffness from developing there and allows non-paralysed muscles to be exercised. It has the great advantage of fitting closely to the hand and is therefore better tolerated than those with 'outriggers'.

10

Elbow orthosis

Conditions for which this is used are:

1. Arthritis of all types.
2. Hemiplegia.
3. Flaccid paralysis, commonly from cervical cord or brachial plexus injuries or neurological conditions such as poliomyelitis or neuropathy such as syrinogomyelia/tabes dorsalis when Charcot joints may develop.
4. Local trauma.
5. Post-arthroplasty either by fascia or metal interposition.

Elbow orthoses are not often used, in general, as their disadvantages outweigh any assistance they may offer.

ARTHRITIS

In arthritis the major use of orthoses is resting the joint and this is achieved by means of a block leather or plastic cylinder or by means of hemi-cylinders for arm and forearm, joined by fixed bars. Such apparatus tends to be inefficient because:

1. The moment arm from the joint to the end of the orthosis in both directions is short, particularly at the upper end where in addition the soft tissue provides poor fixation.
2. Generally no special suspension is provided so the orthosis tends to slide down the arm and cause uncomfortable pressure at the joint. Consideration must be given to simple suspension straps crossing over the shoulder and round the chest.
3. Such a device will limit not only flexion/extension but also pronation/ supination when, commonly, this is not a necessary part of treatment. This unnecessary loss of valuable functional movements is a significant handicap. If fixed the forearm should be some 30 degrees of pronation from the mid-position for optimum range of function when the shoulder can abduct freely. If this is considerably limited or painful, full pronation may be necessary. Because for optimum function the elbow needs to be near a right angle, the arm if unsupported hangs with the shoulder in some extension which can be very uncomfortable.

It is little wonder, therefore, that many patients reject such orthoses and prefer to support the elbow when they can in their coat, on a table or chair arm or in a simple collar and cuff sling.

LIMITATION OF MOVEMENT

An elbow orthosis may provide limitation of movement, for the normal or abnormal range. For example:

1. An articulation can be provided which has stops to limit range to the non-painful area or in a paralytic condition with a rachet articulation which can be fixed at different degrees of extension for different functions (Fig. 10.1).
2. In post-arthroplasty particularly where bony excision has been performed with some interposition membrane or in the salvage of failed endoprostheses excessive abnormal movement needs to be controlled.

HEMIPLEGIA

In hemiplegia, turnbuckle devices to try to stretch gradually a contracture have been prescribed but are largely ineffective. In part this is due to poor mechanical design which allows rotation of the cuffs above and below the elbow. It is mainly due again to the short moment arm and the soft-tissue apposition at the upper end.

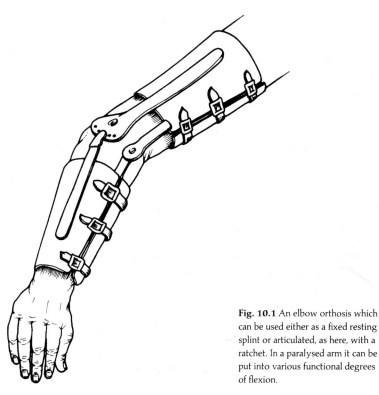

Fig. 10.1 An elbow orthosis which can be used either as a fixed resting splint or articulated, as here, with a ratchet. In a paralysed arm it can be put into various functional degrees of flexion.

FLACCID PARALYSIS

In flaccid paralysis, particularly where extensively affecting a number of other joints, many ingenious devices have been designed with the combined function of controlling joint range and transmitting forces (Schottstaedt and Robinson, 1956). Flexion of the elbow may be achieved by a cable transmission of power from another site, e.g. the opposite shoulder. It is then usual to insert a ratchet into the elbow articulation to maintain it in flexion once the required degree has been achieved to minimize the fatigue that would occur if muscular effort were to be required to maintain the position. This is particularly the case as the mechanical efficiency of such transmitters is low. A further short sharp injection of energy will then unlock the elbow and allow the arm to fall under the influence of gravity.

However, if there is no other available functioning site, outside energy has to be provided. Although several forms have been tried, in general pneumatic stored energy in the form of compressed air has proved most practical. There are still very considerable problems including the replacement of energy source, the achievement of control systems acceptable to the patient, the difficulties of assumption by the heavily handicapped patient and the general cumbersomeness. These problems often cause the devices to be rejected.

Another simpler and more acceptable device is attached to the wheelchair. A metal linkage with ball-bearing swivel joints supports the paralysed or grossly weakened arm; movements of the trunk transmit the minimal forces required to produce important functional movements such as the flexion of the elbow as a necessary part of independent feeding (*Atlas of Orthotics*, 1975; Smith and Juvinall, 1963; Stern *et al.*, 1982).

11

Shoulder

Functionally the shoulder joint itself is an integral part of the scapulohumeral complex. The wide range of movement available in the shoulder joint combined with the movement of the scapular on the chest wall means that the nearest fixed points necessary to the control of movement and position are only to be found on the pelvis and this can make orthoses cumbersome. Fixation around the scapula is more compact but inefficient. This—combined with the increase in internal fixation for fractures and the decline in poliomyelitis for which continuous maintenance of the shoulder in abduction if the deltoid was paralysed was considered beneficial (probably erroneously)—has led to such orthoses being now very limited in use. They are still used for:

1. Acutely painful capsulitis of the shoulder joint. This can be a particular problem at night, substantially denying sleep. In these circumstances the type shown in Fig. 11.1 can be invaluable. It is most easily made of one of the modern plaster-of-Paris substitutes and the essential features are that it curves over the shoulder cap where it is padded to provide suspension, that there should be a bandage incorporated at the level of the humeral neck which is tied around the chest to push the head towards the glenoid, and that distal to this it should be bandaged to the arm. Whilst a resting splint it has the added function of removing some of the tensile stress from the inflamed capsule.
2. Trauma. A similar device is used in humeral fractures and then has the great advantage of controlling rotation of the upper fragment in relationship to the lower. The commonly used hanging cast does not do this and additionally can lead to distraction of the fracture with detriment to union.
3. Neurological conditions: flaccid paralysis—for example, brachial plexus injuries or poliomyelitis—is often associated with considerable further paralysis distally.

    As amputation has often been practised for complete brachial plexus injuries it has been suggested that the function of the prosthesis could be replaced by an orthosis working on similar principles:
    (a) Transmission of energy from a working site, usually the other shoulder by Bowden cable or the use of stored energy.
    (b) A distal attachment into which various tools can be fixed.
    (c) A ratchet elbow attached by cable or by being lifted into position by the other hand.

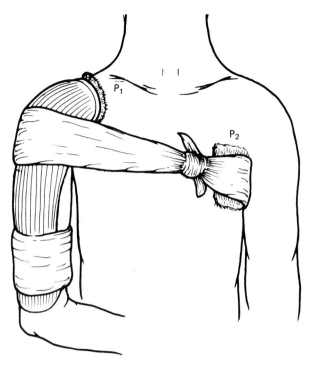

Fig. 11.1 Shoulder orthosis. A plaster or plastic slab is moulded to come over the shoulder joint with a felt pad (P_1) for comfort. A bandage or strap going around the chest incorporated at the level of the neck of the humerus has a felt pad (P_2) stuck to the bandage or strap but not to the patient, which prevents uncomfortable wrinkling in this area. The lower end of the orthosis is attached by a circumferential bandage.

This has resulted in a variety of devices (Fig. 11.2) some with shoulder and elbow function. The problems encountered at the shoulder are mainly concerned with the control of rotation. When the elbow is flexed and the arm even slightly abducted the resultant gravitational force produces internal rotation so that the arm comes to be across the front of the chest in a useless position. This can be overcome but the complexity of the apparatus has led to an extremely high rejection rate. In a valuable review McKenzie and Buck (1978) indicated the criteria for prescription of this sort of device, namely that it should only be provided:

1. If potential for recovery is present.
2. If useful sensation is present (Moberg—two point discrimination of 12 mm or less).
3. If reasonable hand function remains.
4. If reasonably free from pain.

This type of patient often prefers simply to put the paralysed limb 'aside' by putting the hand in his trouser pocket and functioning one-handed with modification of methods and environmental aids suitable to his needs.

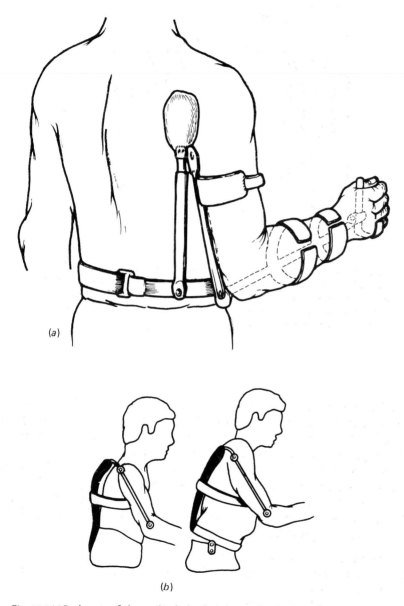

(a)

(b)

Fig. 11.2 (a) Roehampton flail arm splint for brachial plexus palsy. (b) The Rancho Los Amigos Hospital brachial plexus brace has a plastic-moulded corset to which the superstructure is hinged and this enables the patient to lean forward in the writing position without displacement of the shoulder articulation relative to his anatomical joint. This has considerably improved the acceptance of the orthosis which is much more complicated than the schematic diagram here.

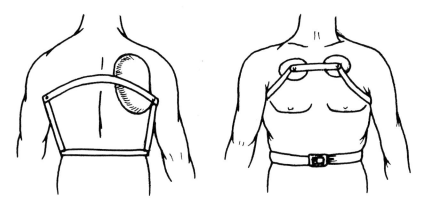

Fig. 11.3 Single scapular support brace. Spring steel encircles the chest with a scapular plate and two anterior supports over the chest wall. This is anchored in place by straps coming down to a strap around the patient's waist.

Serratus anticus palsy can occur in isolation as a result of a viral infection, damage to the nerve supply by trauma or in scapulohumeral dystrophy and may be unilateral or bilateral. Although associated with limited abduction of the shoulder, varying between 60 and 90 degrees, this does not prove to be a major disability for most patients. Changes in daily activity practices often prove more acceptable than orthoses. More of a problem is the 'winging of the scapula' which occurs when the patient undertakes any activity that requires forward pushing. They find it difficult to achieve this with any useful vigour. Orthoses have been designed to hold the scapular to the chest wall and provide a fixed point from which the arm can function (Fig. 11.3). They are of limited value (Johnson and Kendall, 1964a,b; Russek and Marks, 1953; Trulong and Rippel, 1979).

12

Hip orthoses

Orthoses dealing with isolated hip conditions are used for:

1. Congenital dislocation(s).
2. Perthes' disease.
3. Aberrant hip movement in cerebral palsy.
4. Persistent internal rotation of the hip often with upper internal femoral torsion.

CONGENITAL DISLOCATION OF THE HIPS

This is now considered to occur in two forms:

1. That associated with hypermobility of joints.
2. That associated with failure of normal development of the acetabulum.

Associated with hypermobility of joints

This may be generalized and relatively transient, lasting only a month or two; or it may be associated with an inherent tendency to this condition (a rare associated condition is Down's syndrome which can be permanent) and last in the order of 7 years. Because of routine neonatal examination diagnosis is usually within 1 or 2 days of birth. As 50 per cent of such cases recover spontaneously within 5 days, it is reasonable to use orthoses only after this time. The objective of treatment is primarily to maintain the reduction obtained by manipulation. To do this the hips need to be held in abduction, externally rotated and extended. It is important that this positioning should not be exaggerated as this can endanger the blood supply to the femoral head with the development of aseptic necrosis of the femoral head and then early osteo-arthritis in the young adult. Static orthoses, now made of malleable metal covered with leather or latex (von Rosen's splint (von Rosen, 1956) is a classic example, Fig. 12.1) can be kept available in a variety of sizes in maternity and paediatric departments. The metal can provide a problem, as a compromise must be maintained between the ability to mould this on to the patient and the need for it to be rigid enough to maintain the position even with large, strong babies.

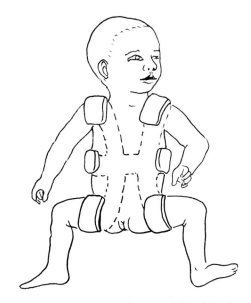

Fig. 12.1 von Rosen type splint for congenital hip dislocation.

The maintenance of cleanliness, skin health and hygiene requires the instruction of the parents to avoid danger of loss of position. Although von Rosen advocated bathing the child with the splint in position, it is usually more satisfactory to train the parents to remove the splint and replace it.

The availability of some movement is thought to be an advantage in maintaining muscular development (although clearly babies can and do use their muscles, pressing against static splintage) and avoiding any danger of aseptic necrosis. The Pavlick harness (Ramsey *et al.*, 1976; Mubarak *et al.*, 1982) is good example of this type (Fig. 12.2) and has the added advantage of being better tolerated both by babies and by parents because the absence of metal framework reduces interface problems, and the design allows toiletting without removal. Abduction and flexion just above a right angle, with an angle between the legs in the coronal plane of never less than 60 degrees, is the recommended position to be achieved by adjustment of the straps. Treatment for 3 months is adequate in this type of congenital hip disease.

Associated with failure of normal development of the acetabulum

As one would expect, early treatment would not necessarily affect the prognosis, and follow-up of these cases has shown that this is the case. This has meant that despite consistent routine postnatal examinations and treatment, the incidence of 'late' cases has not declined. By late it is meant from 1 or 2 months onwards. Treatment then depends on the possibility of satisfactory reduction monitored by appropriate radiological techniques. If that is the case then the use of the orthoses described is possible although the later the diagnosis the greater the tendency to use plaster-of-Paris fixation combined, if necessary with operation.

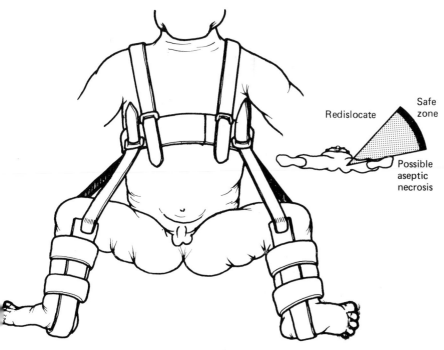

Fig. 12.2 Pavlick harness—inset indicates permitted safe area of abduction range.

PERTHES' DISEASE
(LEGG–CALVE–PERTHES' DISEASE; JUVENILE COXA PLANA)

This is a self-limiting condition with primarily a necrosis of a varying amount of the femoral head, followed by revascularization with healing. During this process the head under the influence of weight bearing would be flattened in all planes. It 'mushrooms' and the congruity between the femoral head and acetabulum is lost with the probability of early osteoarthritis.

The essential cause of the necrosis is still debated. The simplest explanation is of trauma causing thrombosis of arterioles, but it is now apparent that there may be inherent metabolic disorders which predispose to the condition. There is considerable debate as to the correct treatment. Clearly the long-term objective is to reduce the possibility of early secondary osteoarthritis and because of the inherent difficulties in long-term follow-up with appropriate statistical controls, no firm scientific evidence exists regarding the comparative values of different treatments or, indeed, of any treatment. At one time children would be immobilized on a frame in hospital for 2–3 years (Brotherton and McKibben, 1977; Evans and Lloyd Roberts, 1958). Whatever the ultimate value of this, it had serious potential side-effects: namely the psychological, educational and domestic consequences for the patient and family; financial consequences for the health service; and possible adverse permanent physical changes elsewhere in the skeleton, for example knee deformities.

For all these reasons it is now accepted that treatment should interfere as little as possible with the normal life of a patient in this age group. The protagonists of no treatment (other than perhaps a short initial period of bed rest to relieve pain) point to the fact that it needs to be absolutely established that treatment delays the onset of osteoarthritis significantly if the childhood disruption is to be justified. Significant means a perid of 10 years or more. The primary disease normally occurs between the ages of 5 and 9 years and it is known that the later the onset the less chance there is of achieving a normal radiological appearance. Similarly, when first seen the more advanced the condition and the more specific the criteria identified, the poorer the prognosis.

Some progress has been made in prospective prognosis by radiological grading of these cases (Catteral, 1971). This has led to classification into four groups of increasing severity, and no treatment is recommended for groups 1 and 4, as grade 1 will recover without this and grade 4 cannot be helped by any treatment. This approach has yet to be evaluated (Hardcastle *et al.*, 1980). Treatment is now based on some or all of the following principles:

1. That the patient should have sufficient mobility to live at home and attend ordinary school.
2. That as far as possible all weight should be relieved from the femoral head during the cyclic change of necrosis and healing to avoid crushing this.
3. That the femoral head should be put into maximum 'containment' position. In no position can the acetabulum completely cover the femoral head (if it did so no movement of the hip would be possible) but if the leg is placed in abduction and flexion each of 40 degrees with near to full internal rotation (absolutely full rotation is to be avoided as it is thought that this, in tensioning the capsule and blood vessels, could further endanger the blood supply to the head) then maximum coverage is achieved and this acts as a mould to aid maintenance of the sphericity of the head. Furthermore, if movement could occur at the hip joint during treatment then the overall containment would be increased and the moulding would be more efficient.

Relief of compression stress

The relief of compression stress is most efficiently achieved by 'defunctioning' of the leg with bypassing of the hip through a crutch and examples of this are:

1. The Snyder sling (see Fig. 5.10, page 47).
2. The Birmingham splint which combines containment (see Fig. 5.11, page 47) (Harrison *et al.*, 1969).

The problems encountered with attempts to achieve this bypass by means of an orthosis solely on the leg have been indicated on page 46, and clearly the best solution is the patten-ended caliper with a patten on the other shoe. Practical points of this are (a) the avoidance of any possible support of the foot on the affected side; (b) the provision of suspension by means of a band passing over the other shoulder to avoid the discomfort of 'tromboning' occurring during swing–stance–swing; and (c) the provision of better ischial weight support than the ring provides.

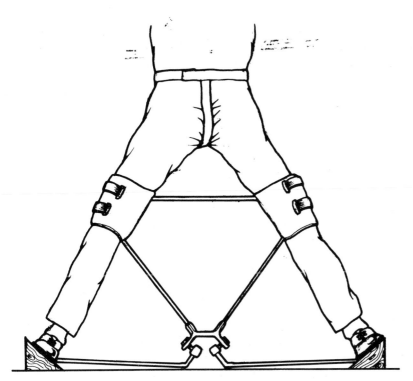

Fig. 12.3 Toronto Perthes' orthosis.

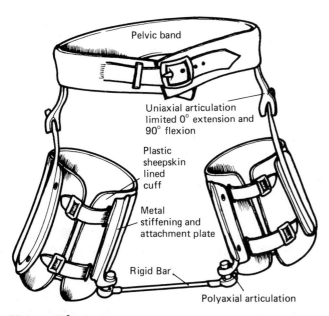

Pelvic band

Uniaxial articulation
limited 0° extension and
90° flexion

Plastic
sheepskin
lined
cuff

Metal
stiffening and
attachment plate

Rigid Bar

Polyaxial articulation

Minimum 35°abduction

Fig. 12.4 Scottish–Rite Perthes' orthosis.

Such devices can only be used in the treatment of unilateral disease which is the common pattern. Not everyone accepts that weight-bearing relief is a necessary part of the treatment and the Toronto (Bobechko *et al.*, 1968) and Newington (Curtis *et al.*, 1974) splints provide containment and movement only (Fig. 12.3). They allow knee and hip flexion to 90 degrees for sitting and the patient can walk in them with a rather high energy consumption and with some environmental damage from time to time as they are heavy and robust. The development by the patient of special sideways techniques of movement are often required with doors of average width. Patients generally use crutches to aid balance.

An orthosis working on some of the same principles but less burdensome is the Scottish–Rite type (Lovell *et al.*, 1978) (Fig. 12.4). This holds the thighs only and maintains the hips in abduction, and some range of this can be allowed. It does not ensure internal rotation and indeed legs always go into external rotation.

All these devices have the advantage of allowing ambulatory treatment of bilateral disease, but no scientific evaluation of their relative effectiveness is available.

ABERRANT HIP MOVEMENTS

Aberrant hip movements occur either as a result of adductor spasm causing 'scissoring' gait or in athetoid palsy where relatively random movements interfere with the child's endeavour to achieve balance and progression.

In the former, orthoses have little to offer as with mild spasm the weight and limitations outweigh the advantages and in the more severe cases inter-face problems and binding of any hip articulations make them useless. However, sometimes after operative intervention a short form of Hip Guidance Orthosis can be useful as a re-educative device. It is in the athetoid patient that most use can be made not only in maintaining the hip movement in the fore–aft pathway, but also in limiting troublesome excessive hip flexion either by appropriate stops in the hip articulations or spring resistance, or by using a full length Hip Guidance Orthosis with free hips and knees and using the weight of the leg sections. Experience suggests that this is the best as longitudinal rotation of the leg is also controlled. The way to provide the required con-trolled 'damping' is one area of potential research. Evidence that any retraining occurs with these orthoses is sparse and they are used to control joint range, therefore.

PERSISTENT INTERNAL ROTATION OF THE HIP

This condition is of two types:

1. The majority where the patient's hip cannot be externally rotated in recumbency with the leg in a position of neutral flexion/extension and abduction/adduction.

2. Where an internal position is assumed on standing but in recumbency full external rotation exists.

Determination of type is a primary step in prescription.

'Twisters'

These orthoses are designed to store energy in either elastic or steel cables tightly coiled in a helical pattern and enclosed in a rubber housing. The energy is supplied when they are put on and is expected to exert an external rotatory tension which will influence bone growth (see Fig. 5.17, page 52). Potentially they are of most use, therefore, in the 2–10 year age group. However, before a child is burdened physically and psychologically with these orthoses, important points need consideration:

1. The natural history and ultimate functional result of this condition. There is a strong natural tendency to improvement although this may occur by compensatory external rotation of the tibia leaving the subject with knees that turn in. There is no evidence that this causes any diminution in gait efficiency, and indeed Tanner (1964) has recorded Olympic winners who have this condition.
2. That the corrective force must be applied to the area of deformity and nowhere else if the production of laxity of the knees or exaggeration of external tibial torsion is to be avoided. To achieve this will require that appropriate moulded knee pieces, either of leather or plastic, embracing both above and below the knee must be added to try to isolate the effect of the corrective force and this increases the complexity of the device and reduces acceptability. Modern operative internal fixation of corrective osteotomies probably makes this the method of choice where it seems that active treatment is necessary. Where the second category of internal rotation is treated such dangers do not exist but consideration of prescription must take natural history and ultimate function into account. Such a device may be of temporary use in training a new posture or whilst awaiting natural recovery in children who persistently trip themselves up.

13

The foot

Treatment of foot conditions has been greatly impeded by traditional diagnostic labelling which has, in fact, little or no clinical significance and illustrates the difference between labelling and classification. 'Flat foot' is a classic example. In this condition, as in many other aspects of the human form, there are wide natural variations, some ethnic and some inherent.

Of all the cases seen in clinics labelled as 'flat foot', perhaps 90 per cent come into this category and the majority are ectomorphs. So arbitrary can this process be that the diagnosis may be changed to cavus feet within a week or two. In the absence of any meaningful diagnosis no rational treatment is possible. As used in this text such terms will mean those conditions for which some criteria of pathology are established.

Feet are the point of contact at which the ground reaction acts and their normal function is to minimize the effects of mechanical stress. This can be subdivided into internal stress and external stress (pressure and shear); the essential mechanical characteristics are indicated in Appendix B.

In pathological conditions either or both of these forms can occur to excess.

To achieve their shock-absorbing function the feet integrate with the mechanisms that exist at the knee and ankle. As the heel strikes the ground at the beginning of stance the knee flexes slightly and the foot is lowered gently to the ground by the eccentric activity of the·quadriceps and ankle plantar flexors, respectively. At the same time, the arch of the foot which has been raised just prior to stance by the active extension of the great toe (which tightens the plantar fascia and supinates the foot) then descends, the foot pronates and this is coincident with an internal rotation of the tibia. At mid-stance the process is reversed with supination of the foot, raising of the arch and external rotation of the tibia.

It is essential to realize that this sequence of events occurs in three dimensions so that the foot is changing in shape both fore and aft and rolling inwards (pronation) and then outwards (supination).

PATHOLOGICAL CONDITIONS

Flat foot

Four types exist:

1. Congenital
2. Hypermobile hyperpronated.
3. Spasmodic valgus.
4. Rheumatoid pronation.

Congenital

This is exceptionally rare and is due to a dislocation of the scaphoid on to the dorsum of the talus. Treatment is surgical.

Hypermobile hyperpronated (Fig. 13.1)

This is associated with some degree of hypermobility elsewhere, particularly in the metacarpo-phalangeal joints of the fingers, the thumb joints, elbow, knees and with abnormally long calf muscles (Fig. 13.2). As this condition improves with age, usually by 7, the objective of treatment is to restore the foot to the normal posture in which it is stable and maintain this until the hypermobility has diminished. If this is not done, secondary changes occur— the calf muscles shorten and the pronation increases further because of the change of the position of the joints in space. The internal mechanical stresses fall on the medial capsule of the mid-tarsal joint which is relatively weak and stretches in contradistinction to the very strong spring ligament which normally supports the midtarsal region (Rose, 1982). Over the years these joints will become arthritic. The effect of these changes is to defunction the shock-absorbing mechanism of the foot. The importance of early efficient treatment for this condition is indicated by the only scientific investigation of the degree of disability in feet conditions—that of Harris and Beath (1947), who found that it was the major foot condition resulting in discharge or down-grading in 3500 Canadian soldiers.

In this situation efficiency of treatment is easy to assess even with the foot hidden in the shoe as correction is always accompanied by an external rotation of the tibia and this can be indicated and measured by attaching a simple pointer to the subcutaneous border (Fig. 13.3). The prescriber may wish to produce either inversion of the foot or supination. The essential difference is that in the former the joints at the bases of the metatarsal rays remain in full extension whilst in the latter they are flexed and the correction is applied only to the hind foot.

Therapeutically inversion suggests that the essential lesion is hypermobility and thus one wishes to hold the foot in the corrected position for a given period; supination that the problem is due to a short or hypermobile first ray (Morton, 1935) and one is trying to stimulate corrective growth. It has been demonstrated (Rose, 1958, 1962) that:

1. Neither supination nor inversion is produced by any form of raise applied to the inner border of the heel.
2. Inversion is produced by a raise applied to the inner border of sole and heel.
3. Supination is most easily produced by a horizontal force applied to the mid-tarsal region.

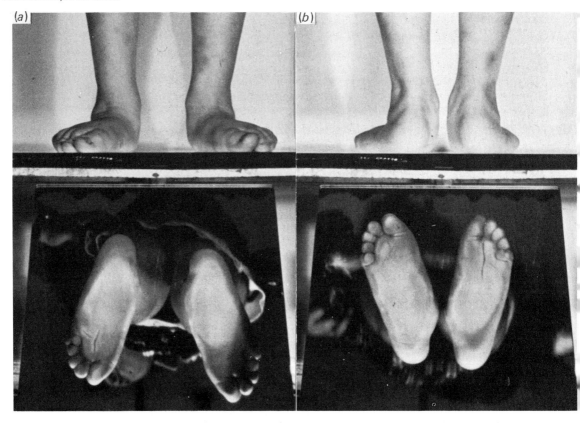

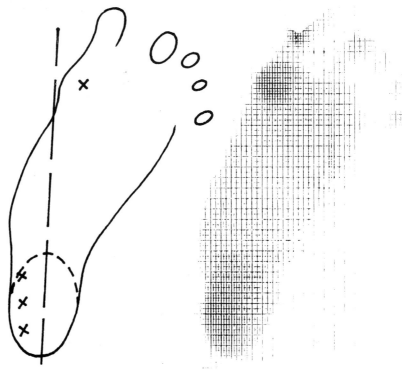

Fig. 13.1 Characteristics of the hypermobile, hyperpronated foot. (a) Reversed internal longitudinal arch, heel valgus, internal rotation of the great toe nail. (b) Mal-distribution of pressure under the sole of the foot along the medial border with an obliterated arch.

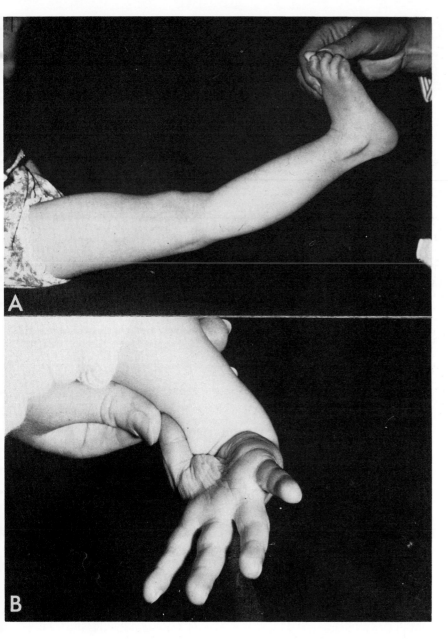

Fig. 13.2 Hypermobility of the knee (A) and thumb (B) associated with hypermobile, hyperpronated foot. Note long Achilles tendon at this stage. This shortens secondarily.

4.   Because pronation is accompanied by an inward rolling (Appendix B) of the os calcis this can be prevented by a wedge placed medially beneath the os calcis always provided that the design is such that this wedge is maintained in position relative to the foot, e.g. Rose–Schwartz meniscus.

Ideally this treatment will be started as soon as the child commences to walk. The foot has the maximum covering of subcutaneous tissue and is most difficult to hold in an orthosis. Experience has shown that the most certain way to obtain and hold the correction is by means of an outside iron and Y-strap.

Consideration of the mechanics of this situation is instructive. The first step

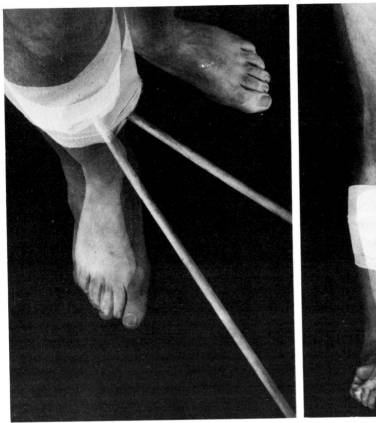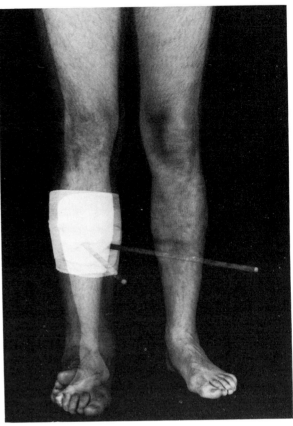

Fig. 13.3 A pointer attached to the subcutaneous border of the tibia demonstrates the rotation that occurs on supination of the foot.

was to ensure that the direction and point of application of the force was correct so that the classic T-strap was modified to a Y thus moving the force from the lower end of the tibia to the medial mid-tarsal region. The average T-strap has no function in this region and is indicated by the gap (Fig. 13.4(a)) which normally exists between it and the strap.

It follows from this change in shape that the two strap arms are now oblique (Fig. 13.4(b)) and not horizontal as in the T-strap. Where these straps encircled the outside iron, resolution of forces meant that the strap progressed down the iron with loss of corrective force. It was necessary, therefore, to pass the strap through a retaining metal loop (Fig. 13.4(c)). Having done this the foot, unless opposed by a third force under the lateral edge of the heel (a reactive wedge), would progress laterally and either cause painful apposition against the outside iron, or eject the spur from its socket. This problem was solved by the use of a Rose–Schwartz insole (see (4) above).

Efficient mechanical attributes for correction were now complete; but it then became apparent that because of these, marked intermittent destructive stress was placed on the spur root where it met the iron and that quite small, fragile children would break the iron once a week. This occurred because it was impossible with a fixed angle to obtain a constant correspondence between the angle of insertion of the spur and the floor-contact heel surface during all

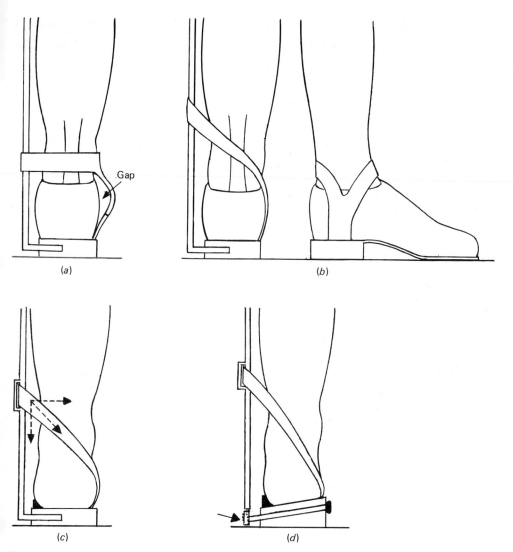

Fig. 13.4 Steps in the design of an efficient outside iron and Y-strap to provide correction in severe hypermobile hyperpronated foot.

phases of gait. The final component of the orthosis, therefore, was a stress-relieving articulation placed at this point (Fig. 13.4(d)), the most successful of these being a comb-hinge.

This orthosis is well tolerated by parents and by infants until they are of school age when, because of the reduction in subcutaneous fat and (very commonly) the improvement in the foot, combined with the need for a less obvious orthosis, it can be changed to a type of plastic insole which derives functionally from the Whitman Brace (Whitman, 1888). This also provides a horizontal force medially on the mid-tarsal region but this is derived from the body weight (Fig. 13.5) which holds the device in the corrective position. It has been called by a number of eponymous and commercial names (Helfet, 1956), none of which vary in principle but many vary in efficiency and com-

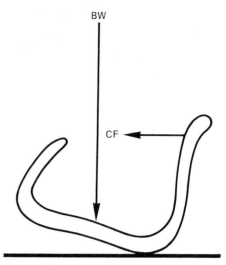

Fig. 13.5 Plastic insole. Body weight, BW is transformed into a horizontal corrective force, CF.

fort. It is best described as a distally extended heel cup (Fig. 13.6). It should be custom made to a cast of the corrected foot and this foot posture is easily obtained and held by the combined use of manually applied external tibial rotation and of extension of the great toe with the patient standing (Fig. 13.7).

Although in these cases extension of the great toe will not normally cause arch rise and supination (and indeed the absence of this has been used as the most important test for pathological flat foot), if the foot is first corrected then it can be locked and held in this position by this technique. It is then relatively easy to build up the plaster slab on which it has previously been placed to form a cast of the corrected foot.

From a negative cast a polypropylene shell can then be formed and this material has sufficient 'give' to produce a well-tolerated device as regards interface pressure.

Commonly, children will develop some thickening of the skin medial to the mid-tarsal region which is painless and which disappears when the need for the insole is past. Parents are often concerned but can be reassured, always provided that the condition is painless.

It is essential that the cast is made weight bearing. It is not always appreciated that the transverse contour of the heel pad in these circumstances is almost square. A similar square section for an orthosis, either for foot or below knee, is important in securing the desired turning of the vertical force through a right angle, which the curved surface produced by casting the non-weight-bearing shape of the foot will not do, itself tending to roll.

Another essential is adequate length. The commercial insert derived from the data given by Helfet (1956) suffers not only from the fact that it comes in standard sizes which are not always appropriate to the patient's needs; but also under the action of the forces generated between the foot and the insert it tends, as do all similar devices, to rotate horizontally, the lateral border moving medially. Since it is short it then presses uncomfortably behind the fifth metatarsal head.

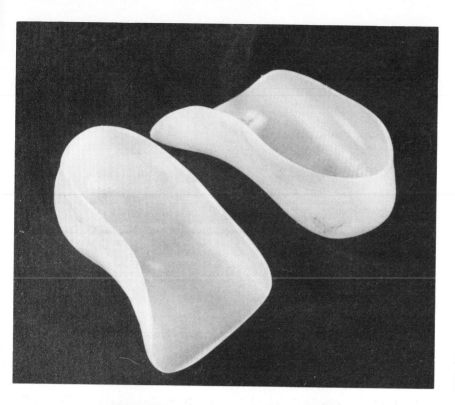

Fig. 13.6 Custom-made polypropylene distally extended heel cups.

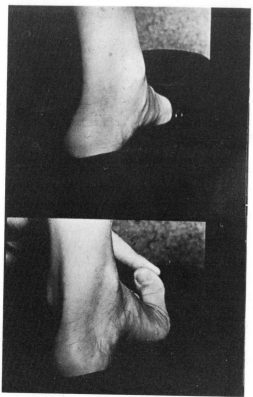

Fig. 13.7 Extension of the great toe causes arch rise and tibial rotation in the normal foot. This mechanism can be used to hold the hyperpronated foot whilst casts are made.

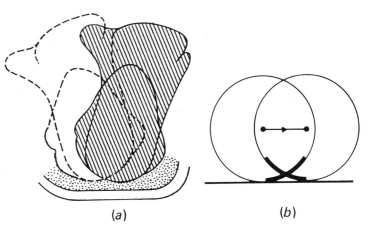

Fig. 13.8 The rolling action of the os calcis from side to side within the subcutaneous tissue and skin in (a) can be compared to the rolling action of a wheel (b).

The inward rolling of the heel of the pronated foot is opposed very efficiently by a wedge placed under the 'wheel-like' contour of the os calcis (Fig. 13.8), as it is in other situations such as the prevention of a wheeled vehicle from rolling down a hill. This is because the wheel, to overcome the wedge, has to rise up on it and this is resisted by the weight, in our case of the body.

A meniscus to prevent inward rolling of the os calcis is ideally shaped in essence as shown in Fig. 13.9, the medial side producing a comfortable efficient wedge and the lateral preventing the heel from slipping laterally away from the wedge with failure of correction. To maintain the two arms in the correct position under the load, the space between is filled with a membrane and this is covered on the underside with an adhesive at the time of manufacture which can be exposed by the removal of a protective film. This alone, however, is not sufficient to oppose the horizontal torsional forces. Displacement due to these is prevented by the addition of two nails driven through the upper surface of the medial wedge and countersunk.

This orthosis has many advantages. Like the distally extended heel cup it can be fitted into shoes or sandals and can be fitted on an immediate outpatient basis. This means that the shoes do not have to go away for an indeterminate period, and this reduces the number of pairs bought by the parents—a considerable financial saving. Furthermore, all internal devices will last the natural life of the shoe, whereas additions to the sole—whether applied to it or inserted as a wedge in various layers—will be subject to wear. In some children in order to maintain correction this may require the parent to provide three pairs of shoes, to allow for renewal of the prescription and transport to and from the works.

External additions to the sole and heel of the shoe are still commonly prescribed. A recent orthotic catalogue showed diagrams of 'some of the more common varieties' and illustrated 18 variants. It is inconceivable that each can have a separate function when the biomechanics are considered and investigated. In general, such wedges must be applied to the sole and heel as indi-

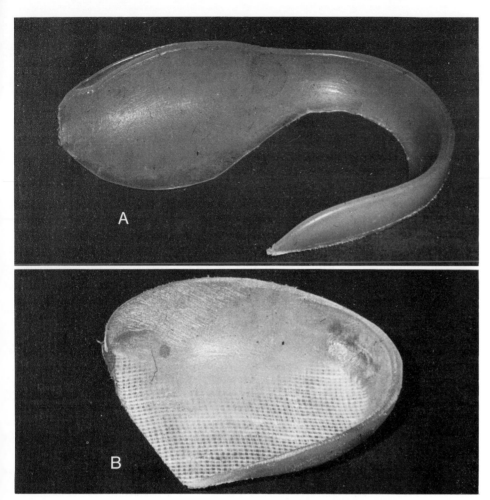

Fig. 13.9 The design of the Rose–Schwartz meniscus to provide a wedge to prevent rolling of the os calcis. (A) Shows the essential components of the meniscus but in (B) divergence of the arms is prevented by a linking membrane.

cated previously, and to be efficient must be maintained consistently in the face of wear.

Spasmodic valgus

This condition, more common in boys than girls, occurs in early adolescence and is heralded by pain and sometimes a limp. It is thought that the primary lesion is in the mid/subtalar joint complex and may be related to a congenital lesion there, such as calcaneonavicular impingement or bar. The foot is in maximum pronation and there may be spasm of the peroneal muscles, but examination under anaesthesia which abolishes this spasm usually shows the foot to be rigid. Before the age of 12 years removal of the bar with stretching of the Achilles tendon (tightness of which often develops as a secondary feature) can allow correction which is maintained initially in plaster-of-Paris and then with an orthosis, either an outside iron and Y-strap or an extended heel cup. In those cases where correction is not possible the device will be supportive and reduces the abnormal internal stresses. If continued for a number of years the foot often becomes symptom free and has a useful function. If either internal or external stresses produce symptoms then operative correction becomes necessary.

Rheumatoid pronation

Rheumatoid arthritis commonly causes hypermobility of joints which may be accompanied by collapse of osteoporotic bone and rupture of the tendon of the tibialis posterior muscle (which when intact with increased activity of the muscle can provide some protection against pronation). If the latter occurs the foot may undergo a sudden and dramatic postural collapse. If the foot remains correctable it can be stabilized mechanically and held by iron and Y-strap or an extended heel cup with no interface problems. Where this is not possible the device becomes again supportive and because the disease causes thinning of the skin and subcutaneous tissue with reduced vascularity interface pressure and shear is poorly tolerated. Lining the heel cup with thin foam layers may help in this respect but the resultant heat retention can cause excessive discomfort.

Cavus feet

Distinction has to be made between high arched and cavus feet. Again one has the problem of natural variations. Two main pathologies can be distinguished:

1. High arched pronated feet.
2. The progressive neurogenic foot accompanied by clawing of the toes, inversion of the foot and sometimes with vascular and sensory deficiencies which predispose to trophic ulceration.

High arched pronated feet

Because of the considerable pronation with marked shift of the ankle medially in relationship to the heel this can be confused, even by an experienced prescriber, with the flat foot which also has this degree of ankle shift. It is this type of foot in which again rupture of tibialis posticus occurs which can cause considerable disability often in middle age. Again if fully correctable it can be dealt with by one of the orthoses already described. To achieve this correction very adequate stretching of any shortening of the Achilles tendon will be a vital preliminary step. When used supportively and particularly if tendon rupture is present, interface problems may cause rejection particularly as these patients are otherwise fit and try to be very active.

Progressive cavus

It is now generally accepted that progressive cavus is neurological in origin even when the defect cannot be absolutely identified. It is then probably due to minor congenital abnormality of the nerves of the cauda equina. Spinal Dysraphism (James and Lassman, 1972) is the next most serious condition and is due to tethering of the nerve roots to the spinal canal by abnormal bands. When the normal disproportionate growth occurs in the first few years of life between spinal cord and spine, the cord cannot rise up in the canal and traction on the nerve roots occurs. This commonly leads to the quite rapid development of a unilateral cavus of marked degree and can, in some cases, go on to more extensive paralysis. Early identification and appropriate spinal operation is most important to limit the degree of disability. Even so, the foot may require orthotic and operative treatment.

There is no evidence that any orthosis can prevent the progression of the pathological cavus foot with its neurogenic muscle imbalance. In general, the orthotically treatable problems are:

1. Both pressure and shear stress under the metatarsal heads subsequent upon the increased angle of inclination of these to the support surface, which may be aggravated by a shortness of the triceps surae and of a relative equinus consequent upon the cavus itself. Where other neurological features are present, such as sensitivity or circulatory changes, the situation can be complicated by ulceration.
2. Inversion instability which can both reduce the efficiency of gait and shift and the area of pressure laterally under the foot.

Orthotically for (1) the highest level of care and supervision is required with the provision of a multi-layer thermoplastic insole for relief of pressure and a rigid soled shoe for relief of shear. For any serious degree of cavus this means inevitably an orthopaedic boot made on orthodox principles. (2) can only be dealt with orthotically when modest in degree because in marked deformity the coronal moment (consequent upon the ground reactive force which acts during stance phase and can be considerably higher than body weight) either cannot be resisted by an orthosis or the interface pressure is intolerable.

Footwear makes the situation (2) much worse. Fig. 13.10 indicates the

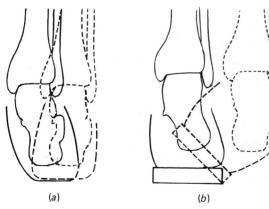

(a)   (b)

Fig. 13.10 Anteromedial tomographs of the ankle barefoot and in a shoe, normal posture and supinated into an unstable position. (a) The instability only slightly increases in the barefoot position owing to the outward roll of the os calcis keeping it under the tibia. (b) In a shoe it is greatly increased, as is the movement of the ankle within and without the support area.

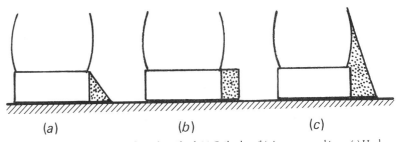

Fig. 13.11 Useful forms of 'floated out' heel. (a) Orthodox. (b) A wrap-round type. (c) Heel brought up to help support the upper.

change that occurs on supination of the bare and shod foot. In the former, because of the mechanics of the lateral heel roll, the moment about the subtalar joint axis is relatively small compared with that in the shod foot. This is because the heel elevates the subtalar axis and increases the moment arm whilst at the same time producing an edge fulcrum, laterally displaced. Interestingly, the shoe upper normally reaches only to the subtalar joint and has little or no effect, therefore, on the stabilization of this in any circumstances. This confirms the need to persuade patients with lateral instability to wear boots; fortunately fashion changes have made acceptance of these easier in recent years.

Furthermore, it will be seen that the higher the heel, the greater the moment and the narrower the heel, the less stability; a combination of conditions which occurs commonly with the female shoe or boot. Increased stability will come with broadening of the support area by the floated-out heel, a very undervalued orthosis (Fig 13.11).

In more severe cases this can be combined with an appropriate medial short iron and lateral Y-strap with the modifications previously noted to secure maximal mechanical effect. The problem of foot movement within the shoe may defeat the orthotic objective and this can be avoided by the coincident use of a distally extended heel cup made in the standing position with the foot corrected as far as possible.

Painful heel

The precise nature of this condition is not known, but what is known is that it is not related to the bony spurs that can be seen on X-rays so that both operations designed to remove these and insoles designed to remove pressure from the area of the spur are extremely disappointing. It has also to be recognized that in some intractable cases painful heel can be an early sign of systemic rheumatic disease and in particular ankylosing spondylitis and Reiter's disease. It is not then relieved without appropriate general treatment. Most cases, however, appear to be in the nature of an area of inflammation under the medial weight-bearing area of the os calcis adjacent to the bone. In this area the plantar fascia is continued over and closely applied to the periosteum to join with the Achilles tendon. The best way of relieving pressure is to roll the os calcis inwards without applying pressure to the tender area. The heel meniscus

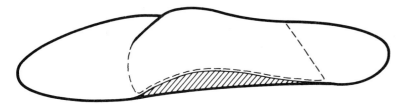

Fig. 13.12 The Rose–Parker insole (convex wedge). This is a firm Sorbo-filled insole higher on the medial side than the lateral.

is not suitable for this purpose, therefore, and it may be best achieved by using a convex wedge (Rose–Parker insole, Fig. 13.12). The wedge is made of firm rubber foam and has proved very reliable. In intractable cases a below knee rigid plaster cast applied in the non-weight-bearing position thereby retaining the uncompressed dome of subcutaneous tissue can be walked on without pain. It would seem that the compressed soft tissue acts hydrodynamically to relieve pressure from the tender area; after at least 6 weeks it can then be re-placed by the insole worn at least until this wears out.

Metatarsalgia

Metatarsalgia is pain from any cause in the forefoot area. Two types exist:

1. Consequent upon mal-distribution of weight sharing under the metatarsal heads.
2. Morton's metatarsalgia consequent upon the formation of a neuroma on a digital nerve and this may be secondary to damage to the blood supply to this. It commonly occurs in the 3/4 interspace, can be burning in character and may be intermittent, occurring when the neuroma gets pressed upon by the internal structures of the foot when this is in a particular position. It can then be relieved on occasions by manipulation but may require opera-tive removal of the neuroma. It may be relieved by a metatarsal dome or convex wedge but this can only be determined by trial and error.

A mal-distribution of weight can affect one or more heads. In the normal foot it has to be emphasized emphatically that there is no transverse arch under the metatarsal heads and that the weight is normally distributed under all the metatarsal heads more or less equally. Some modest inequalities are, as in all areas of the body, compatible with entirely normal function. Prominence of the metatarsal heads in the sole is closely related to clawing of the toes and this to the function of the plantar fascia (Fig. 13.13).

When a single toe has a fixed flexion at the proximal interphalangeal joint (and it is commonly the second which forms a hammer toe) when standing the proximal phalanx is into full extension and the metatarsal head is forced below the level of the others. In weight bearing this head is then heavily overloaded

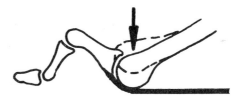

Fig. 13.13 The fixed clawing, at the proximal interphalangeal joint (arrow) tightens the plantar fascia and forces the metatarsal head downwards through the subcutaneous tissue. The dotted line indicates the level of the other metatarsal heads.

with consequent callosity formation, thinning of the subcutaneous tissue and diminution of the shear relieving function. By inserting an insole carrying a metatarsal dome behind the callosity some load will be bypassed from the metatarsal shaft to the contact surface. Relief can only be temporary as the intervening soft tissue atrophies; a higher dome is then required and the process repeated, but clearly this cannot be done endlessly. The essential problem of fixed flexion at the proximal interphalangeal joint remains.

In circumstances like these it is the duty of the orthotist to discuss the problem with the prescriber. An added disadvantage of the use of such domes is that where one or more toes are clawed callosities are often present over the proximal interphalangeal joints as the deformity cannot be accommodated in the shoe depth. The orthosis then pushes the toes even harder against the upper. It can to some extent be helped by the use of a three-quarter insole rather than a complete one. This then has to be anchored in place by a tack in the heel area.

It is also clear that if some degree of clawing of the toes is present the extension of the toes which normally occurs passively at the last third of stance (the toe rocker) will worsen the situation and an orthotic change to diminish or remove this will be helpful. A metatarsal bar is recommended.

A metatarsal bar

There are two practical problems with this. If the sole of the shoe is not sufficiently strong, the bar will indent the shoe, becoming ineffectual and uncomfortable. To prevent this it may be necessary to insert a metal or rigid plate throughout the length of the sole. The second problem is the placement of the bar. Traditionally it is said that this should be behind the metatarsal heads and it is often placed at the posterior edge of the sole. It is said that this 'transfers the weight posteriorly and off the metatarsal heads', but this does not accord with any mechanical theory. The load remains under the heads and may be transferred to the floor more posteriorly but this has no beneficial effect on the foot. If, on the other hand, the object is to reduce extension of the toes Fig. 5.31 (page 65) shows that it is better placed forward. In practice it is always better to incorporate the bar in a rocker sole as this avoids problems which can occur if the bar catches on a projection, the accelerator pedal of a car for example. If the foot condition is associated with any equinus then the heel must be

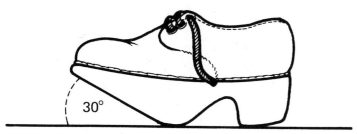

Fig. 13.14 Mandatory rigid sole contour to avoid both pressure and shear stress. To achieve this with toe comfort it is often necessary to raise the sole and heel.

raised appropriately to correct pitch to avoid increasing the pressure under the metatarsal heads.

Such form of footwear modification also has the advantage of transferring the toe rocker function from the foot to the footwear–ground interface, not only eliminating the shear stress at the metatarsal heads but also allowing a nearer normal gait pattern diminishing stresses on other leg joints. This is particularly important in widespread disease such as rheumatoid arthritis. The correct sole contour has been determined by Brandt and others (Fig. 13.14) and the validity of this has been demonstrated in the treatment of neuropathic ulceration in leprosy, diabetes and spina bifida.

FOOTWEAR

The problems of footwear are complex and emotive. Some basic understanding of these is essential particularly as patient satisfaction can be extremely difficult to achieve in some cases. In a recent survey (Bainbridge, 1979) whilst 82 per cent of the recipients of surgical footwear were satisfied, of the 18 per cent dissatisfied, 6 per cent were 'very dissatisfied'. There are three areas of dissatisfaction:

1. *Footwear*—30 per cent experienced some discomfort from poor fit initially and in 12 per cent this persisted even with wear. Twenty-nine per cent could not put on their footwear or only with difficulty, 19 per cent disliked the colour or style and 14 per cent (21 per cent of child wearers' parents) were dissatisfied with the durability.
2. *The rate of delivery*—Inordinate waiting times can mean that the available pair becomes worn out before the new ones are ready in adults, and in children the new pair being outgrown before it is delivered. In the above survey 25 per cent were delivered within a month, 66 per cent in 2 months and 14 per cent in 4 months.
3. The number of pairs available at one time.

Although it is recognized that surgical footwear is a major source of orthotic problems, 63 per cent of patients saw the doctor only once and that was for the initial prescription; 24 per cent were seen additionally on completion of the footwear; and only 6 per cent were seen at the preliminary fitting stage. Too often surgical shoes are ordered in the mistaken belief that being made to measure they can cure all problems, including failed foot surgery. The likelihood of failure is greatly increased if the prescriber and orthotist have no mutual understanding of the specific aims in each individual case and do not completely understand the essential problems of producing satisfactory footwear, both commercial and surgical. This fundamental feature is common both to prescriber and to orthotist. Whilst at first sight it might seem that a perfect cast of the foot should produce a perfect last on which to mould the shoe, there are two major reasons why this is not so:

1. The dynamic changes in the shape of the foot during walking require a compromise not provided by a static cast. The arch rises and falls, the foot pronates and supinates, the plantar fascia becomes prominent in the sole medially and allowance has to be made for this, particularly in higher heeled shoes.
2. The need to hold the shoe on the foot during both stance and swing. In late stance as the heel of the foot comes off the ground it has to take the shoe with it and requires, therefore, some 'waisting' of the upper in this area. During swing the design must prevent the shoe falling off or more often becoming displaced, so that at the beginning of stance there is no unpleasant 'socketing' of foot in shoe which rapidly produces blistering.

To some extent the situation is easier in the grossly arthritic foot where the patient will progress slowly, with a short step length and little or no dynamic change in foot shape. In such cases casts used as lasts can be reasonably successful, particularly when allied to a rigid rocker sole. The most troublesome problem here is likely to be oedematous swelling which must either be controlled by an elastic stocking (which rheumatoid patients with hand problems may find impossible to put on independently) or make some allowance for it. In this case the heel grip is particularly important. Modification of the plaster cast to make a last (rectification) requires skill and experience combined with a detailed knowledge of the patient's specific problems and this must include:

1. A clear statement of the objective of the prescription; for example, is it to provide relief from internal or external mechanical stress or both? Is it simply to provide a covering for a foot which cannot be accommodated in commercial footwear either because of the foot shape itself or because when insole or insoles are provided for another purpose the combined foot and orthoses cannot be covered in any other way.
2. A satisfactory method of transmitting the complex data required from orthotist to maker. Many firms now provide complex measuring charts. These can be supplemented by plaster casts even though these have limitations as has been indicated. In a very deformed foot a plaster cast is mandatory but too often it is found that the orientation of the foot, and therefore the cast, to the ground is omitted. The result may fit the foot well, but be unstable if the support area (sole and heel) is not in normal contact with the ground when the patient stands. The situation is most important when a raise is also required for then the turning moment producing instability is increased as are the quite unnecessary and gratuitous strains on the foot and ankle. In the most difficult cases time and money is saved by direct contact between maker and patient.

In general two forms of surgical footwear are now made:

1. Those of orthodox design in which the upper is stitched to the sole.
2. Those made of thermoplastic material, often vacuum formed to a suitably modified plaster cast of the foot.

The first are most suitable for vigorous patients, particularly those in employment with adverse working conditions such as the presence of water or oil, but do require the patient to have good manual dexterity to put them on. The latter are more suitable for indoors and limited outdoor wear in the less active patients, often suffering from rheumatoid arthritis and often requiring very simple closure methods such as Velcro fastening flaps because of considerable hand and arm deformities.

Marked shortening of a leg has largely disappeared in new patients attending orthotists. This is because of: (1) surgical treatment, both preventive and restorative; (2) the disappearance of some diseases that produced severe shortening, notably poliomyelitis; and (3) the increased use of prostheses in congenital lesions.

Where compensation for leg shortening is required, the orthodox procedure has been to do this by the insertion of cork either between the upper and sole or incorporated into the upper of footwear of orthodox design. For reasons of both weight and lateral stability the maximum raise is in the region of 30 cm (12 in). The presence of a raise removes the flexibility of the shoe and it is therefore important to provide an appropriate taper from the level of the metatarsal heads to the toe (or, confusingly, toe spring in footwear terminology) to allow a comfortable toe rocker action (see Fig. 5.32, page 66).

For robust individuals requiring a higher raise a patten may be used. Because of the weight and unsightliness this is now almost wholly restricted to use as a temporary device in patients wearing a patten-ended caliper on the other leg. In developing countries, however, it can be valuable because of its simplicity of manufacture and wear, and its robustness in adverse weather and ground conditions.

Where a caliper is used with a raised shoe thought needs to be given to the point of insertion of the tube. Technically it is convenient to insert it into the leather heel rather than the cork raise but from the point of view of the complex linkage between the ankle and rotation of the spur, the tendency to forward movement of the ankle relative to the caliper is minimized by having this inserted near to the foot.

In such considerations as these it must be emphasized that patients who have fully mobile joints elsewhere are often able to modify their gait pattern to compensate for these situations and either position will be equally acceptable, but where there are constraints at other joints the optimum positioning of the tube may become very important for comfortable gait. An alternative solution is to insert a square spur into the heel and provide an articulation corresponding to the axis of the ankle joint.

FASHION AND THE SURGICAL SHOEMAKER

Ladies' shoe fashions remain the surgical shoemaker's unsolved problem. A good example of this difficult area is shown with shoe raises. For many years the orthotist tried to persuade patients with one leg shorter than the other that a separate style raise was not really all that bad and did not too much detract from the overall appearance of the individual.

New patients had been known to shed tears about having to wear this particular adaptation. Overnight, platform soles became the fashion and young patients started pleading for incorporation of raises to both shoes to emulate the current trend. The fashion circle has since turned and the raise is once again considered to be disfiguring.

The real problem encountered almost every day is the lady with a broad splayed forefoot, hallux valgus, prominent metatarsal heads, corns on most of the toes and a bunion. This patient often totters in through the door wearing a pair of elegant patent leather court shoes, with a high unstable heel. Opening comments revolve around how many pairs of shoes are in the wardrobe, none of which are wearable, and how she has resisted surgical shoes for years. She realizes that she can no longer walk as well as she used to and hopes that a pair of shoes can be made which will look the same as the ones she is wearing. Clearly they can, but will not fit and will not relieve her problems. The request for a court shoe poses particular problems. A well-fitting shoe of this type, if the foot is not to come out of the heel during the second part of stance, relies on a longitudinal compression between the heel cup and the metatarsal area pressing against a rather tight vamp (the ill-fitting shoe achieves this by wedging the toes right up into the front of the shoe). Any form of surgical shoe must transfer the forward hold to the mid-tarsal region using laces, straps or elastic there. This should always be explained to the patient before measurement is commenced to avoid problems of acceptance later. Indeed, the ideal situation is for the patient to see a specimen of the type of shoe that will be provided.

A patient should, however, be encouraged to select colour and design to choice, and the orthotist and shoemaker should explore every avenue within the compass of the correct design to satisfy the wishes of the individual.

14

Below knee orthoses (AFO)

These are far and away the most common orthoses for the lower limb being supplied perhaps 100 times more often than the others put together, excluding footwear. The variations in design are innumerable but these are all changes rung on the following main types.

(1) *Metal and leather*—They have a leather-covered metal calf band with one or two metal side bars or a posterior bar. The bars may be rigid or a variety of spring depending on the function and may be inserted either within the shoe as a sole plate or into the heel. The insertion into the shoe is no new concept and was commonly used early in this century but fell into disuse because of the simplicity and cheapness of spurs inserted into a heel tube. The axis of rotation of the spurs does not correspond with that of the ankle and in movement this causes the side bars to move relative to the ankle and shank (Fig. 14.1) a situation often well tolerated by many patients. However, it is an increasingly common practice to insert the ends of side irons rigidly into the heel by means of a plate with joints as for the knee which are dealt with later (page 155). With rigid bars ankle-joint movement can be controlled by springs or stops of various design but it is always an advantage to have some built-in element of adjustment so that optimum function can be achieved by tuning during use.

(2) *Plastic*—Which are most often contoured to fit the limb closely and to be inserted inside the shoe (Lehmann, 1979; Yates, 1976). Variations in ankle movement and degree of resistance to movement is derived both from the shape and from the characteristics of the plastic used. They are lighter to wear

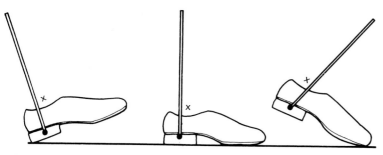

Fig. 14.1 Geometry of the movement of the axis of the ankle joint (X) relative to the heel inserted side iron.

than the metal and leather, cosmetically more acceptable (often both visually and aurally) but need more attention to shoe fittings and take slightly longer to get used to.

(3) *Hybrid devices*—Combining some of the structure and function of both.

Biomechanically classified, these orthoses have the following functions:

1. To limit movement range—normal or abnormal, complete or partial.
2. To stabilize the foot.
3. To exert a knee control function.
4. To relieve longitudinal or lateral stress.

LIMITATION OF MOVEMENT RANGE

Used in:

1. Neurological conditions causing either flaccid, athetoid or weakly spastic paralysis.
2. Primary diseases of the muscles—flaccid paralysis.
3. Spastic paralysis.
4. Associated valgus or varus deformity.
5. Arthritic conditions of the ankle.

Lesions of neurological conditions

The neurological conditions causing flaccid paralysis are in the main those causing lower motor neurone lesions from the anterior horn cells downwards. These include such conditions as anterior poliomyelitis, multiple sclerosis, traumatic and congenital lesions of the cauda equina, nerve root compression from prolapsed intervertebral disc and peripheral nerve lesions. It can occur in the upper motor neurone lesion of the spinal cord due to trauma or congenital abnormality, i.e. myelomeningocele. Associated spasm is variable in incidence.

Orthotically an important subdivision is the presence or absence of sensation, both from the point of view of potential interface problems but also, in the higher lesions whether proprioception is present. In its absence the patient will have difficulty in appreciating the position of the limb in space and the foot will then approach the ground in varying positions during walking. This can be a major cause of failure to improve gait by this means both in stroke and in multiple sclerosis, and this should always be assessed prior to prescription by the prescriber or the orthotist taught by him how to do this.

Primary disease of the muscles

In primary disease of the muscles, such as dystrophies and myopathies, there will obviously be no sensory defect.

Spastic paralysis

Spastic paralysis is caused by disease or trauma of the upper motor neurones, mainly those in the brain, and includes head injuries, tumours, and neurovascular incidents such as thrombosis of cerebral vessels.

Important subdivisions are those patients with impaired skin sensation and the type of spasticity, whether very slight or vigorous, and in particular the reactive response to stretching of the affected musculature. Sometimes this will be negligible whether done slowly or fast, whereas in others only slow stretching will maintain a relaxed state. Then the practical implication is the need for dorsi-flexion restraint to avoid provoking this spasm during the second part of stance. This variation makes the use of spring-loaded orthoses a matter of considerable judgement. Certainly the degree of exaggeration of the spasm by stretching the affected muscle should be tested by the orthotist both by fast and slow stimulation. Where there is any sign of a brisk response, all springs must be avoided.

Forces that modify foot posture can be threefold, although all do not necessarily act at once:

1. Gravity.
2. Where only part of the musculature working across a joint is affected, the relatively stronger groups will deform in the direction of the resultant dominant force. Whilst this may be obvious, the discrepancy may be so subtle as to escape clinical recognition on formal examination and only becomes apparent as an end result. This is particularly the case where there is a high level of paralysis and sensory loss as in spina bifida. Here the residual muscular activity may be reflex in type and not under voluntary control. Any muscle inbalance is highly efficient in deforming whereas the best orthoses are relatively inefficient; whilst these may delay the rate of increase they seldom, if ever, prevent it. This is an area where long-term surgical–orthotic integration is essential.
3. The ground reaction. An inverted foot, for example, striking the ground on the outer border can be forced into further inversion by this. An orthosis, a boot with appropriate insole and external re-alignment, can move this reaction to a more stable position and reduce the total deformity (Fig. 14.2). It goes without saying that here, as with all shoe inserts, the bottom of the insert should match the contour of the shoe if the effect of the shoe is to be transmitted to the leg (Platts *et al.*, 1979).

Initially the overacting muscle, particularly if normal, will allow the deformity to be corrected but gradually a contracture occurs (i.e. shortening of the available excursion) and prevents correction. The nature of this contracture varies. In normal muscle it can usually be stretched but in spastic muscle and even in the acting muscle in poliomyelitis changes occur that prevent this, and the remedy is surgical.

In considering the function and secondary effects of these orthoses both the geometry and the forces acting are important. It has been said, for example, that in a dropped foot as foot clearance is one important orthotic objective the degree of dorsi-flexion is irrelevant provided that it is well above a right angle. Consideration of the geometry of this situation shows that there is an opti-

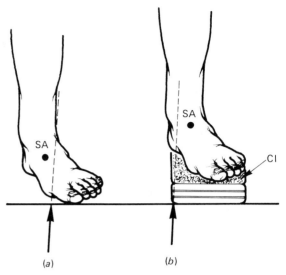

Fig. 14.2 (a) Ground-reaction on the barefoot produces an eversion moment about subtalar axis (SA). (b) With an appropriate cradle insole (CI) and heel support to match, this can become an inverting moment.

mum angle for clearance (Fig. 14.3) and this can be easily demonstrated by standing on one leg and dorsiflexing the foot. Above a right angle the leg is relatively lengthened. Of course, foot clearance is a complex interrelationship of many joints, including the spine. There is no advantage in making this more difficult. There may be more serious consequences as indicated in knee control function when the control exerted can be quite disastrous.

The forces acting are identified by the use of the free body diagram at all stages of gait and in both planes (see page 11). At heel strike there is a considerable moment deriving from body weight which if it acts in an unconstrained way will produce a foot slap with disturbance of the gait rhythm and increased impact under the forefoot. Normally this is optimally controlled by the dorsi-flexors working in an eccentric fashion and clearly it is an important function of the orthosis to reproduce this as far as possible. If it is done with a spring the strength of this can be moderated relatively simply, if sometimes somewhat crudely. When this relies on the interrelated properties (material and structural) of a plastic orthosis the situation may be more difficult.

The normal contour of the posterior leg does usually provide a reasonable product but not if the curves are reversed. In Fig. 14.4(a) this was caused by oedema in a long-standing poliomyelitis; it was necessary to reduce this by bandaging the leg for a time before it could be used as a mould by which to produce the desired mechanical effect. If in an endeavour to reduce the plantar flexion resist the area behind the Achilles tendon is narrowed, the mechanical effects are complex and can, under stress, produce unwanted torsional effects on the foot. Again, the specification can be modified not always in a controlled way by the 'flow' of the plastic during casting when it thins at inappropriate areas. Quite apart from the commercial advantages and speed of supply, these are both reasons for the use of prefabricated devices which are produced by pressure die casting.

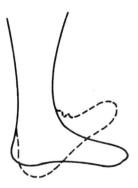

Fig. 14.3 Relative lengthening of the leg that occurs with calcaneus deformity.

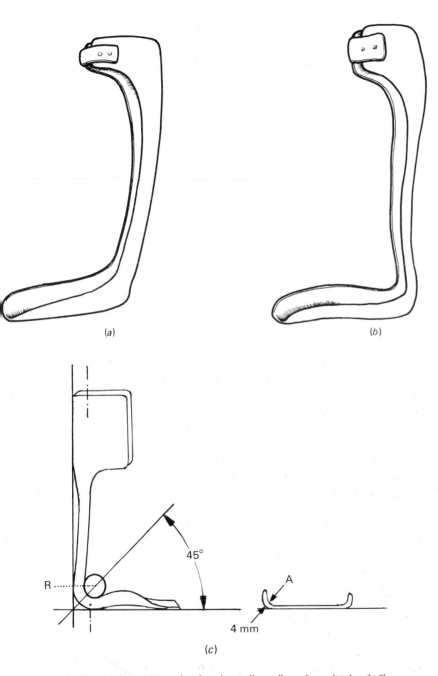

(a)   (b)

45°

R

4 mm

A

(c)

Fig. 14.4 (a) Shape of plastic AFO produced on chronically swollen poliomyelitic leg. (b) Shape of AFO after appropriate period of bandaging. (c) Criteria given for the production of Ortholen AFO:

1. Radii (R) to be equal medially and laterally.
2. A line projected from the centre of radius to its lowest point should form an angle of 45 degrees with the ground.
3. The radius will vary from 13 to 25 mm depending on size of AFO.
4. The edges (A) may need material removed to produce a thickness of 4 mm. It is said that if these points are observed no breakage will occur.

In considering the forces, some important points are:

1. Forces around the upper end of the orthosis and the placement of this. It should be as high on the leg as is compatible with knee flexion. If put over the middle of the calf the moment arms are shortened and the applied force substantially increased whilst the available area of application of this is reduced, increasing the pressure stress on skin and underlying tissues. Furthermore, the application changes from the posterior aspect to the front band which is often inadequately padded and secured. In some of the more heavily handicapped patients where opening of this band in the second half of stance can bring walking to a stop and may even cause a fall, Velcro is insufficient and should be replaced by a modern, easily fastened buckle free from sharp points.

2. That in plastic devices the buckling that occurs during the end of stance can give rise to pressure over the Achilles tendon or a widening of the heel which may, depending on the configuration of the curves in this area, cause unwanted twisting of the foot. The double below-knee iron with a foot-drop spring or the foot-drop stops do not suffer from this problem as they allow automatic adjustment in this respect. This situation can be complicated by the internally generated forces from the triceps surae; for example, whether deriving from voluntary controlled activity as in poliomyelitis or the involuntary action of spasm not always associated with sensory feedback. It may require an appropriate rocker sole both to minimize internal stresses and to improve the smoothness of gait.

Practical problems arising from these factors have resulted in the design of plastic orthoses in which the articulation activity is divorced from the main material and structure and is replaced by the insertion of a metal or plastic joint (Fig. 14.5). In complex problems this has the considerable advantage of the

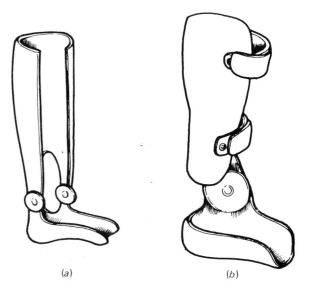

(a)   (b)

Fig. 14.5 Articulated plastic AFO. The articulation can be either double (a) or single (b).

orthotist being able to adjust one element of the function without affecting others, which would otherwise alter unpredictably.

Another factor that affects function is the wear and distortion of the device. A good example of this is the use of foot-drop stops to resist plantar flexion. When new they totally prevent plantar flexion whilst allowing free dorsi-flexion during the last third of stance. At heel strike the normal plantar flexion moment, already considerable deriving from body weight, may increase by spastic reflex extensor thrust from the triceps surae. Inevitably the stops either bend or loosen at their attachment to the heel consequent on the high impact forces. At this point they may become less efficient relying for their plantar resist on the leather strap which commonly runs from one iron to the other and passes round the heel upper (Fig. 14.6).

Although consideration has largely been given so far to plantar flexion resist, excessive dorsi-flexion (either passive or active) can be a considerable handicap. In effect, the patient then walks on the relatively small support area of the heel with reduction in extrinsic stability (see components of locomotion, page 22) and this is very important in widespread paralysis. Additionally, the ground-reaction vector is modified adversely in relationship to the knee (Fig. 14.7) With reversed foot-drop stops the shoe can be made to position the foot

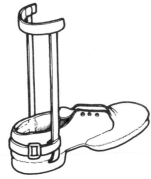

Fig. 14.6 Double below-knee iron with square socket and posterior strap which commonly and inefficiently takes over the plantar resist.

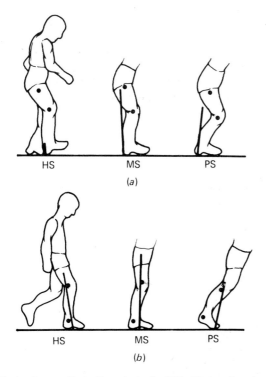

HS   MS   PS
(a)

HS   MS   PS
(b)

Fig. 14.7 (a) Tracing from a patient with cerebral palsy (CP) with excessive calcaneus deformity. HS = Heel strike; MS = mid-stance; PS = pre-stance. (b) Normal. Note that in the normal condition the vector passes forward along the foot as the knee progresses in space so that the moment about the knee is nil or small. In the CP case the moment is always adversely flexing.

correctly (always provided that the dorsi-flexors are not contracted), but again the high level of stress in the second part of stance will soon produce distortion and the posterior strap is less effective because of the narrowing of the heel upper at the upper edge.

If plastic orthoses are used they need to be of the solid ankle type and this will impose modifications on the gait pattern which may be tolerated depending on the pattern of handicap. A spina bifida patient provided with these increased her speed from 70 m/min (225 ft/min) to 76 m/min (250 ft/min) whilst her heart rate fell from 200 to 180 beats/min, indicating an improvement in gait efficiency. Much more importantly from her point of view, she could now stand still for the first time, and her capability to walk a distance increased over six-fold.

Valgus or varus deformity

Where there is associated valgus or varus deformity with flaccid paralysis this occurs at the subtalar and mid-tarsal joint and the mechanics which obtain in the hypermobile flat foot are in general applicable except that an internal constraint may exist in regard to available range of movement. Inversion normally has a large range whilst eversion is small. Conditions causing problems with orthoses are generally concerned with inversion (supination), although the everted foot (pronated) may need to be relieved of painful internal or external stresses. The inverted foot produces a small support area only down the outer border which is further reduced in the presence of equinus. This reduces the balance capacity of the patient, already often impaired considerably. In the absence of marked spasm or contracture, corrective forces can be applied by means of:

1. An outside Y-strap pulling up to a retention loop on an inside iron (the mechanical advantages of this over a T-strap have been indicated; see Fig. 13.4, page 129).
2. Supplementation by the heel being 'floated' laterally. This puts the ground reaction as far laterally from the axis of the subtalar joint as is possible and provides the best everting moment (see Fig. 14.2). This combination ensures that the foot contacts the ground initially in the best obtainable position and that the forces during stance tend to maintain the correction. When spasm or contracture is present a disadvantage of this form of orthosis is that the foot can tend to deform within the shoe. Whilst an extended heel cup may then be used to try to prevent this, commonly the interface pressure cannot be tolerated or the spasm will displace the foot from the insert and/or shoe.

Practically it has been said that if the orthotist cannot attain the correction he needs with his hands, then an orthosis is unlikely to succeed and the prescriber must be informed so that he can consider methods of serial stretching and/or operation prior to the use of the orthosis.

Plastic AFOs can be modified to control the foot by bringing the foot piece up the inner border of the foot. The relationship between the structure so produced and ultimate function can be complex particularly when the internally generated forces of spasm are considered.

Arthritic conditions of the ankle

In arthritic conditions of the ankle in flaccid paralysis when as a therapy to relieve pain the most efficient immobilization of the foot–ankle complex is needed, plastic orthoses are very satisfactory if made in two overlapping sections (Fig. 14.8) as used at the Forrest Hill Hospital, South Africa (Craig and van Vuren, 1976). However, they must as always be combined with a correctly shaped rocker sole and regard must be paid to the knee function. Experiments have established that in pantalar (i.e. of ankle, subtalar and mid-tarsal joints) stiffness a position of 10 degrees calcaneus deformity is ideal because it allows optimization of the sole contour much more easily than does equinus. The resultant orthotic–shoe combination is at a right angle to the shank.

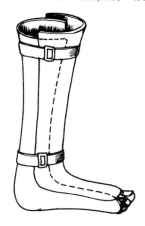

Fig. 14.8 The most efficient orthosis for immobilizing foot and ankle, an overlap type made either in block leather (Forrest–Hill) or in polypropylene.

STABILIZING THE FOOT

The use of below knee orthoses to stabilize a mobile deformity, usually pronation, has already been discussed (see page 127).

CONTROL OF THE KNEE

Knee control function can be beneficial or adverse and functions either by holding the ankle at a right angle or by modifying the relationship of the ground-reaction vector to the axis of the knee joint.

Holding the ankle at a right angle

Orthoses that hold the ankle at a right angle in cases of calcaneus deformity in mild cerebral palsy where there is no contracture or marked spasm in the hip and knee flexors certainly improve standing posture, the subject being straighter and taller (Fulford, 1978). In walking, improvement occurs if the necessary compensatory options are present in other joints.

Modifying the relationship of the ground-reaction vector to the axis of the knee joint

Normally this is maintained near to the axis throughout the stance phase, moving forward along the foot as the knee progresses forward in space, the angle with the ground varying appropriately (see Fig. 14.7). Particularly where there is weakness of the quadriceps as in muscular dystrophy, an equinus produced either by a mild contracture of the Achilles tendon or an orthosis is very beneficial as this puts the ground reaction forward in the foot (see Fig. 3.5, page 24) and produces an extensor moment at the knee supplementing quad-

Front   Back

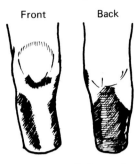

Fig. 14.9 Areas of toleration for pressure in a below-knee amputation stump. These are the areas on which weight should be concentrated in an orthosis.

riceps function. Conversely, if for any reason a calcaneus deformity is produced either by an ill-advised lengthening of the tendon or by use of an orthosis in this position, at heel strike post-operatively the shank will move forward immediately, unopposed by effective action of the triceps surae and carrying the knee into flexion. The situation is even worse with an orthosis, for then the shank will be forcibly rotated forward as the foot goes on to the floor and the knee again destabilized.

RELIEF OF LONGITUDINAL OR LATERAL STRESS

Orthoses that relieve longitudinal stress reduce weight bearing substantially. This owes much to the development of the so-called 'patellar tendon bearing socket'. In fact, transparent sockets have shown that load is distributed over a much wider area than the tendon (Fig. 14.9). In orthotics there is a practical problem not encountered in prosthetics, namely that, except in very exceptional cases, the socket has to be made with an opening to allow the foot to go through. This means that the closure design must be very efficient and remain so under the considerable stresses of usage as in the quadrilateral socket used in the long leg brace. Reference has already been made to research to establish the efficiency of KAFOs for this purpose (see page 44). Similar work has indicated the ideal criteria of this orthosis (Davies *et al.*, 1974; Lehmann *et al.*, 1971), namely:

1. Rigid closure of socket with a 10 degree knee flexion.
2. Fixed ankle at 7 degree dorsi-flexion.
3. Rocker sole and stiffening plate.
4. Heel clearance 6.5 mm (5/8 in).

The usual form is a plastic socket combined with metal side bars, and a very rigid fixation of these by some form of 'fish plate' to a boot which is mandatory (Fig. 14.10).

The orthosis has been recommended for:

1. Short term (up to 6 months):
   (a) Very comminuted os calcis fractures.
   (b) Post-operatively after fusion of the ankle.
   (c) Chronic heel pain resistant to primary treatment.
2. Long term:
   (a) Chronic neuropathic ulceration of the heel area to aid healing.
   (b) Neuropathic arthropathy, e.g. Charcot's disease, to diminish further destruction.
   (c) Ambulation pain in gross arthritis of the ankle–foot complex.
   (d) Delayed unions of fractures, particularly when associated with infection.

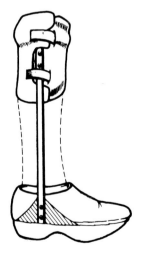

Fig. 14.10 Patellar tendon bearing brace. Note fishplate and rocker sole.

15

Long leg orthoses (KAFO)

The functions of these orthoses are:

1. To relieve weight partially or totally from the hip. These have been dealt with and come within both the KAFO and HKFO depending on whether they are extended above the hip (see page 117).
2. To relieve stress within the leg. Longitudinal stress is a direct result of weight bearing and lateral and torsional stress indirect.
3. Stabilization of the knee:
   (a) In sagittal plane—flexion, recurvatum.
   (b) In coronal plane—valgus, varus.
4. To limit movement completely or partially within the knee.
5. To combine with some functions of the AFO.
6. To exert a hip control function.

RELIEF OF STRESS WITHIN THE LEG

The technical challenges of achieving this have been indicated within the leg (see page 44) (Lehmann *et al.*, 1970b; Lehmann and Warren, 1973); relief may be used for:

1. Treatment of delayed union of fractures of the femur or tibia and fibula.
2. Reducing the interface forces required to decrease partially correctable deformities in the sagittal or coronal plane. For example, an otherwise mobile knee lacking 25 degrees extension will require a force to be applied to the knee as shown in Fig. 5.12 (page 48) to maintain this position. It will be seen that this is related to the weight borne by the limb. If this is reduced so is the interface force in direct proportion. Similar principles apply to valgus or varus angulations. Such reductions will reduce discomfort in patients both with sensation, and in those without the dangers of skin breakdown.

Because of the mechanical characteristics, these orthoses are least able to resist lateral stresses and in the valgus/varus situation it is particularly useful to reduce this even if the longitudinal stresses within the side bars are increased. Conversely, of course, if the KAFO is bent sideways to accommodate valgus or varus, longitudinal stress will be efficient in increasing the angulation of the orthosis and rendering it ineffective. A narrow band or a ring top is then mandatory as is reinforcement of the knee area as shown in Fig. 15.1. Torsional stress relief depends on an upper end which as far as possible prevents any rotation at this level and must, therefore, be a well-fitting quadrilateral socket. Where this is not so and the knee is held straight (thus eliminating any rotational stress relief at this level which normally occurs in the knee flexed some 5 degrees), the torque stress and movement could be increased at the site to be protected, a fracture of the mid-shaft of the femur, for example.

STABILIZATION OF THE KNEE

Stabilization of the knee, particularly the prevention of flexion collapse during walking where the quadriceps is totally, or considerably weakened is the basis of the common traditional long caliper or brace. As has been indicated (see page 23) given ideal circumstances with full extension or slight hyperextension of the knee the orthosis only functions periodically during walking, usually when going down a slope or on rough or irregular ground. In general it relieves the patient from concentration on their mode of walking and prevents occasional unexpected falls. The interface pressures are low. This means that there is a wide tolerance in design. A simple ring or band top placed somewhere in the upper thigh region, poorly aligned articulations, comparatively heavy and with spurs fitting into the heel of the shoe can be acceptable to some patients and on occasions preferred even when a trial of more modern, cosmetically superior splints has been tried. In considering long leg brace design a number of general factors need elucidation:

1.   Weight.

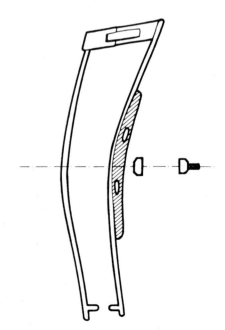

Fig. 15.1 A long leg brace (KAFO) bent to accommodate and support a valgus knee will require strengthening with a lateral plate welded at right angles as shown if it is not to be distorted itself by the forces generated in the knee during walking and standing.

2. Alignment of hinges.
3. Lockable joints.
4. Freely moving hinges.
5. Lower-end attachment.
6. Upper-end design.
7. Fixation at knee level.
8. Stabilization in valgus/varus plane.

Weight

In general the lighter (compatible with safety and reliability) the better but, related to gait efficiency, the problem is not a simple one:

(1) *The amplitude of the body centre of mass through space* means that the total body weight has to be lifted recurrently and not all the energy thus used is returned. This energy deficit is increased by a heavier orthosis but calculation suggests that this is relatively very small.

(2) *An important element in forward progression is the inertial energy released at the end of swing*—As inertia is related to weight this propulsive energy is increased by the heavier splint. This is offset by the proportionately greater energy cost of initiating swing and on balance, therefore weight in this respect makes little difference.

(3) *Much more important is the natural periodicity of the leg pendulum* which is simple in type if the knee is locked. This determines optimum cadence and this is unrelated to absolute weight but is directly related to the distance of the centre of mass of the limb plus the splint from the hip. It is the distribution of weight which determines this and most efficient gait is produced if both limbs are the same in this respect. Where there is a freely moving knee joint a compound pendulum is produced and this is more complicated. In general the same principles apply to periodicity but the inertial extending relationship between shank and thigh will carry the limb forward to full extension for inherent stability at heel strike. In this case the centre of mass of the whole leg and of each segment should match the other limb.

Alignment of hinges

Hinges are commonly used for sitting only and are locked during walking and only rarely unconstrained during gait. There are two elements of alignment:

1. Alignment of the axis of one hinge with the other.
2. Alignment of the orthotic and anatomical axes in all planes. The knee does not have a single fixed axis but as the knee bends the axis moves in space—the instant centre pathway (Fig. 15.2).

Alignment of the axis of one hinge with the other

Malalignment makes flexion of the knee difficult and in marked malalignment may make the range for sitting inadequate and/or as flexion occurs the lower

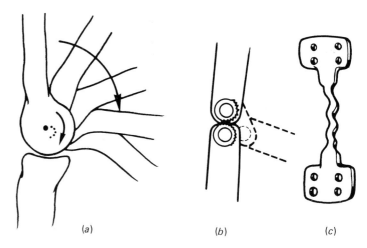

Fig. 15.2 (a) Although knee flexion is regarded as a hinge action, the axis of the hinge moves in space as the knee is flexed. (b) To correspond with this, geared polycentric joints have been designed to accommodate this, but for reasons given they are not always necessary. (c) The plastic polycentric joint is used in cast bracing.

segment will twist in relationship to the other. Where the device is spur ended and the shoe loosely fitting this may be tolerated but can cause interface problems in the closely fitting plastic orthoses. Obviously, this situation will also cause increased wear and the development of troublesome laxity. An orthodox caliper with hinges needs a rigid calf band to ensure simultaneous locking of both hinges and avoidance of twisting stresses on the joints. The function of this band allows clearance between it and the calf, but this must be checked in all positions of flexion to avoid the complications indicated in the next section, or pinching of a fatty pad at the lower popliteal region due to the band being too high on the side bars.

Alignment of the orthotic and anatomical axes

If the orthotic hinge is above or in front of the anatomical axis, on knee bending the thigh band will slide down toward the knee. If this sliding is prevented as when the top is joined to a body brace, the patellar band will press into the leg, a matter of potential danger where the skin is insensitive (Fig. 15.3). If the orthotic axis is behind or below the anatomical axis the thigh band will slide upwards, possibly causing groin discomfort or if this is resisted the calf band will press into the underlying tissues if snug fitting in the standing position. By bending the knee with the caliper fitted, these points can be checked and adjustments made.

Hinges usually have the axis of rotation placed eccentrically within the hinge structure in order to avoid unsightly prominence of one component or associated wear of clothing (Fig. 15.4). More complicated and therefore more expensive and less robust polycentric joints have been designed to match the movement of the orthotic axis more closely to that of the knee but are not

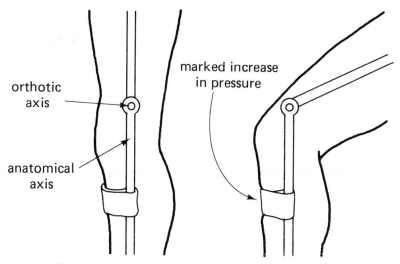

orthotic
axis

marked increase
in pressure

anatomical
axis

Fig. 15.3 Change of relationship in orthotic and anatomical axes in sitting.

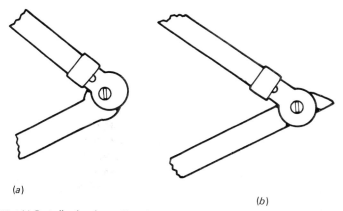

(a)

(b)

Fig. 15.4 (a) Centrally placed axis of knee hinge produces a troublesome prominence on flexion. (b) The eccentric hinge avoids this.

much used, as the tolerances of fit usually accommodate the otherwise inevitable slight discrepancies of axes on flexion.

Lockable joints

When stabilization is secured by using the knee joint locked, it is desirable that unlocking to sit should be an easy, one-handed function with automatic relocking on standing. This should be entirely reliable, and accompanied by an easily heard 'click' as a feedback for the patient. There are a wide variety of such joints but they are, in principle, most commonly of two types:

1. A spring-loaded ring catch joint which is basically a tube of appropriate matching section which slides over part of the articulation (Fig. 15.5(a)). It is difficult to join two such locks together without interfering with their function and often they therefore require a two-handed release.

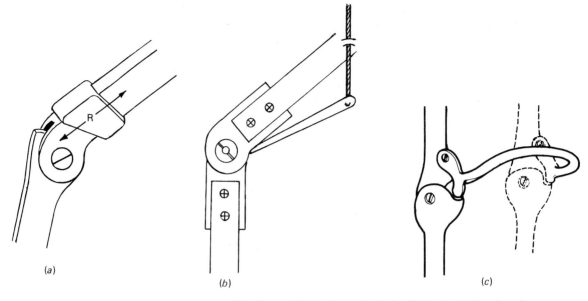

Fig. 15.5 (a) Ring lock. The ring (R) slides down to lock when the knee is straight and may be spring loaded to do this automatically. (b) A ratchet or bail lock (when joined together, a bar lock). (c) Whilst theoretically only one locking joint is necessary, for mechanical and safety reasons two should always be provided.

2. A rachet or bail lock. In extension the pawl of the lock engages in the rachet and is held in the locked position either by springs incorporated in the locks or more reliably and robustly by joining the two pawls together with a bar posteriorly (thus forming a barlock which can be opened with one hand) and attaching to the middle of this bar a broad elastic which is attached at its lower end to the calf band (Fig. 15.5(b)).

Variations include cords and/or rods to bring the control higher in the leg and sometimes in the heavily handicapped patient bringing the bar anteriorly to avoid a dangerous interference with the posterior mechanism by the edge of the seat. This problem tends to occur in patients wearing two such braces, who are overweight and have a considerable struggle to get upright from a wheelchair.

Freely moving hinges

Because of the ability of patients with paralysed quadriceps and normally aligned knee with either full extension or some hyperextension to walk satisfactorily on level ground without any orthosis at all, attempts have been made to design long leg braces with freely moving hinges which would protect the wearer against instability in all circumstances. As any type of long leg brace has obviously no function during swing the free hinge allows knee flexion at this time to aid limb clearance and reduces the need, if the limb is of equal length, for such energy-costing manoeuvres as circumduction and/or pelvic 'hitching'. It has been suggested that set-back knee joints can be of help because the ground-reaction vector then passes in front of the articulation and produces an extensor moment. The solution is not so simple. In the majority of this type of brace very little loading passes through the brace and in this case it is the relationship of the vector to the knee axis which is all important. This will depend on two factors, position of the knee axis (itself dependent on degree of hyperextension) and orthotic techniques to move the vector forward. Two methods can be used:

1. Advancing the heel contact (Fig. 15.6) which produces a modest advantage.
2. Orthotically producing an equinus and hence primary toe contact. This achieves a greater shift but a relative lengthening of the limb with greater centre of mass rise and increased energy cost.

Of course, if the knee has a little flexion deformity some compromise can be made if the brace is made very substantially weight bearing by means of a quadrilateral socket and it is then that the position of the orthotic axis becomes relevant. It has to be recalled, however, that in this situation the upper end will move upwards during swing but the brace will tend to move downwards and suspension must be secure.

Experimental models produced include the Otto Bock four bar linkage and the UCLA (University of California Los Angeles) functional long leg brace. The latter uses a quadrilateral socket, set-back joints, wedge heel and a hydraulic damping device at ankle level which allows some slight damping of plantar flexion after heel strike to avoid foot slap and much more marked damping of dorsi-flexion which helps keep the vector forward in the first third of stance. Additionally, movement above a right angle is totally prevented. These free-knee devices are contra-indicated if there is:

1. A 10-degree flexion contracture.

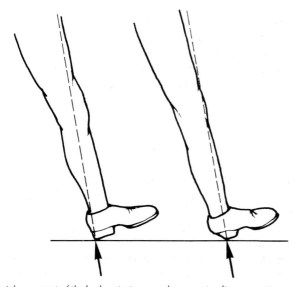

Fig. 15.6 Advancement of the heel contact can produce an extending moment around the knee.

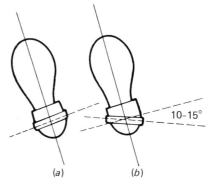

Fig. 15.7 (a) Correct placement of a spur tube to the heel. (b) For reasons given, the oblique placement sometimes recommended is ineffectual.

2.   A valgus deformity of the knee.
3.   Absence of hip extensors which also produce an extensor moment about the knee as a secondary effect.
4.   A need to use the orthosis frequently on sloping or irregular ground.

These types are considerably more expensive than the locked-knee type and are not likely to come into service until some way is found of designing the kind of mechanism used so successfully in above-knee amputations. A considerable space exists to accommodate this. The problem in an orthosis is to fit a suitably slim mechanism to the sides of the joint.

Lower-end attachment

Lower-end attachment has the same characteristics as those used for below knee orthoses but one additional point must be mentioned. It has been said that in order to provide a normal 'toe out' alignment of the foot that the attachment to the heel should be placed at an oblique angle (Fig. 15.7). This is unnecessary and ineffectual, the turning out of the limb being initiated at the hip level. With a looser fitting type of upper end there is sufficient tolerance for the adjustment to be made unconsciously but when a quadrilateral socket is used in which rotation cannot occur the heel socket must be correctly aligned with side bars or with the knee in a plastic type.

Conversely where for any reason, such as muscle imbalance, in-toeing occurs, modifying the angle of the tube does not cure it.

Upper-end design

The upper-end design largely depends on whether or not the orthosis is to be maximally weight relieving. As has been indicated, the quadrilateral socket (see page 44) derived from prosthetics where all weight bearing is total is the ideal solution (Lehmann and Warren, 1973). Forces applied to the upper edge of the front of a thigh band have been estimated during paraplegic gait and shown to cause intermittent superficial blood flow occlusion but also considerable shear which can cause abrasions or sores. Skilful experienced fitting is essential in these devices. Variants, such as the moulded lace-up leather top made to a plaster cast (bucket top) are very substantially less efficient. Importantly, it has been shown that a plaster cast of the upper thigh does not produce an ideal shape and leather gradually deforms under the influence of sweat and heat, whilst lacing is mechanically less efficient than the tongued opening of the plastic socket. It has its use, however, as for example in an elderly patient with an un-united fracture of the mid-femoral shaft. The block leather can then be prolonged downwards to provide an element of total contact and control.

Fixation

Fixation of the orthosis at the knee level should be minimal, as should all orthotic fixation compatible with function and safety. The fastening of unnecessary buckles and clips adds up to a considerable time penalty for the heavily handicapped in particular, and even more importantly can reduce their independence. The mechanics of this situation have been considered in relationship to degree of knee flexion (see page 48).

In the dynamic situation in the straight knee, experiments have been conducted to calculate the shear force tending to produce backward subluxation of tibia on femur (Lehmann *et al.*, 1976) and these have confirmed the importance of the patellar band in all phases of stance in reducing the stress on the knee ligaments. In these conditions it is evident that the commonly supplied knee cap (see Fig. 5.14, page 49) is unnecessary and patient reports and clinical experience confirms this. Made of plastic with a suitable padding and an easily closed clip on the outer end they are safe, quick and easy to close (see Hip Guidance Orthosis, page 186). Interface pressures estimated in paraplegic walking (which causes the highest stresses) were found to be sufficient to occlude superficial blood flow and were even higher if the bands were not carefully adjusted, not only to provide a large contact area but also to use it. These pressures do not cause clinical problems because the brace functions intermittently throughout ambulation and they are, therefore, applied also intermittently. This is an important contrast to the flexed knee where in stance they are continuous as well as being much higher. Knee flexion contracture of greater than 5 degrees is an indication for consideration of surgical release.

Stabilization in the valgus/varus plane

Stabilization of the knee in the valgus/varus plane depends on two factors:

1. Correctibility of the knee alignment.
2. Stability of the intrinsic bony structures of the knee when this is achieved.

As these deformities are often accompanied by angulation of one or more articular surfaces (Fig. 15.8) stability is not achieved by restoration of normal

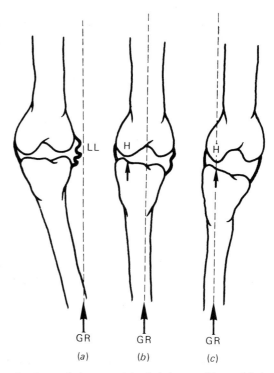

Fig. 15.8 (a) A valgus knee with distortion of the tibial plateau and laxity of the lateral ligament (LL). (b) Alignment of the leg secured, there will still be a turning moment about the present hinge (H) and the lateral ligament may still have some laxity. If this is the case (c) will stabilize about the hinge (H). GR = ground reaction.

alignment and some degree of 'over-correction' may be required if the advantages of stabilization, namely low interface pressure on the valgus or varus strap are to be achieved. In rheumatoid arthritis associated with poor skin tolerance this may be extremely important. If this is not done the orthosis becomes a supportive one.

LIMITATION OF MOVEMENT WITHIN THE NORMAL KNEE RANGES

Hugh Owen Thomas devised his splint initially for the complete limitation of movement during bed treatment of bone tuberculosis and when he judged this stage to be completed would cut off the far end and turn the side bars into the heel of a boot to make a walking caliper.

Whilst this disease has largely disappeared in the UK for the present, its tenacious capacity to reappear must not be forgotten. It still flourishes in many parts of the world where modern plastics are prohibitively expensive whilst simple blacksmith and leather skills are available in every village, and this simple, robust and easily repairable device comes into its own for prolonged complete immobilization. It can be used as an adjunct to the treatment of septic infections once the acute stage has been treated with appropriate antibiotics and surgery if necessary. This will quite commonly result in some initial loss of a few degrees of extension with a cold knee and a painless range beyond this. Joints can then be provided to limit full extension and hence reduce trauma to healing tissues. Similar situations may exist with degenerative and rheumatoid arthritis where there is often some limitation due to some 'squaring' of the condyles.

HIP CONTROL

The Craig-Scott brace (Heize, 1967; Lehmann, 1979; Scott, 1980) was produced to exert hip control in traumatic paraplegia. Whilst it has other desirable features the objective is that 'the centre of gravity of the patient can be used to provide control of balance during standing'. In principle it is, therefore, analogous to the posture instinctively assumed by the patient suffering from muscular dystrophy of the Duchenne type (see Fig. 2.3, page 11) in securing intrinsic stability. The patient does not fall backwards as extension of the hip is prevented by the natural constraints—the strong anterior ligaments—and he or she reduces the handicap of weak hip extensors by maintaining a posture both standing and walking with the body centre of mass behind the hip joint. This is only possible if there is no flexion contracture of the hip and there is a mobile lumbar spine producing a lordosis. Because of the intact sensation these patients can monitor this situation with accuracy by intrinsic feedback, an advantage denied to the traumatic paraplegic. To make the situation as efficient as possible in paraplegia the following design features are provided:

1. Strong rigid brace construction.
2. A reinforced rigid shoe joined to the side bars with a rigid fish plate with an inbuilt adjustment for optimum dorsi-flexion. If one considers the body outline it is apparent that this is required to produce extrinsic stability.

Additionally to facilitate doff and don a single rigid pretibial band with easy locking is provided just below the knee, and spring-loaded bale-lock knee hinges are provided for sitting. The axes are set back 6.5 mm (5/8 in) from the line of the side bars both to avoid sharp protruding edges when the knee is flexed and also because in this position when standing the forces tend to extend the joints and this means that the unlocking requires little force. If at this time there was a tendency for joints to flex the unlocking would be hard and would engender wear which in turn threatens the rigidity of the system.

The problem of such a system compared with the hip guidance orthosis is that it requires the available joint extension noted above. Also, very importantly, any ground irregularity can cause an inertial continuation of trunk movement with loss of intrinsic stability. This has been a considerable problem, often reducing patient confidence and substantially limiting the supply of KAFOs to those with muscular dystrophy.

MODERN DESIGN

The advent of plastics has lead to considerable and rapid changes in orthotics which have sometimes been made without regard to two important and related factors:

1. That the principles of functions are unchanged.
2. That the materials used have to be appropriate to the identified mechanical problems.

Used appropriately, plastics represent a valuable and now permanent part of orthotics. One such advance has been the so-called 'cosmetic caliper' (Tuck, 1974; Yates, 1976) (Fig. 15.9). Undoubtedly there has been a considerable improvement in cosmesis but this label obscures its other advantages and the biomechanical implications. 'A plastic conforming caliper' would seem to be somewhat better terminology. Two thermoplastic materials are at present in common use, polypropylene and high-density polyethylene (Ortholen) which are hand moulded or vacuum formed at an appropriate temperature on a plaster cast of the lower limb made with the patient lying supine with the limb held in the position of greatest correction consistent with comfort. Particular care is needed in aligning knee and foot. The thigh and below-knee sections are made separately, the latter usually of greater thickness than the upper because of the mechanical demands, and are then joined by appropriate metallic side bars incorporating locking hinges. The lower section is inserted into the shoe and can be modified depending on the function demanded of it, as in the AFO.

Advantages of modern design

1. Lightness; about half the weight of the orthodox type.
2. Cosmesis. Conforming as it does with no outside projection at the heel, covered with a stocking it is very unobtrusive visually and is also free from the various noises that can arise during walking with other types. Wasting of the calf can be concealed with plastic foam which can be appropriately 'skin' coloured as can the plastic itself. Importantly also the foot piece can be made to insert into normal commercially made shoes to allow women in particular to have a much wider choice of these and the ability to use different shoes throughout the day without each pair needing to be modified.
3. Can be cleaned and hygiene is improved.
4. The inserted foot piece has some movement relative to the shoe so that there is an element of compensation and stress relief on the orthosis on walking over rough terrain.

In general this orthosis is suitable for cases without, or with easily correctable, deformities in which the function is stabilization. Whilst claims have been made for some degree of weight relief (BRADU Report, 1979) it cannot be weight bearing as it cannot fulfil the design characteristics already noted as necessary. Also, it has mechanical weaknesses deriving from the attachments

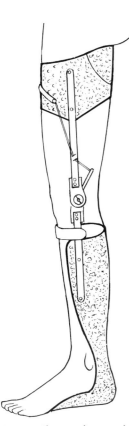

Fig. 15.9 Plastic conforming caliper ('cosmetic caliper').

of the metal side bars to plastic components and from the curvature of these which produces a weaker mechanical structure than the straight side bars of the older type.

Where there is slight valgus or varus deformities which are completely correctable, interface problems can be reduced by a degree of weight relief from a quadrilateral socket but this causes stress to the orthosis itself. The conformation produces its own problems.

As it is customary to cast for this brace with the patient lying the resulting form will not correspond to that of the leg when weight bearing; for example, in regard to the change in shape of the heel pad. Heat retention and sweating may be troublesome in some patients as will large changes in size from postural oedema. Growth in children may dictate frequent changes of orthosis, as adjustment is limited. Some slight modification in shape is possible in polypropylene with a heat gun and in Ortholen by hammering as this has a certain degree of ductility similar to metal.

FUNCTIONAL FRACTURE BRACING (CAST-BRACE)

It is convenient to discuss here a therapeutic area in which orthotists, physiotherapists and occupational therapists are becoming increasingly involved, and it is convenient to deal with it in a separate section. Its label derives from the objective of maintaining a normal limb function as far as is practicable during fracture healing.

It has long been known that fractures with little or no fixation have a very rapid union rate but the price to be paid is shortening and malalignment in all planes. Attempts to avoid these complications by orthodox plaster casts has led to a much higher proportion of delay or non-union combined with gross muscle wastage and joint stiffness that requires prolonged rehabilitation, recovery from which may never be complete. On the other hand, rigid internal fixation whilst producing perfect repositioning and allowing joint movement so removes the stimulus to bone union that this may be inadequate and eventually under repeated mechanical stresses the internal fixation will break and non-union result.

Functional bracing (Meggitt *et al.*, 1980; Sarmiento and Latta, 1981) is a middle course applied not as a primary treatment but at the stage where the general guidelines are:

1. Minor movements are painless.
2. No shortening on longitudinal compression.
3. Angulation produced is elastic and self-correcting.
4. Shortening should NOT exceed 6 mm (1/4 in) for the tibia and 12.5 mm (1/2 in) for the femur.

Retention of fracture position is dependent on:

1. Mechanical holding principles including three-point fixation and the soft tissue hinge.
2. Hydrodynamic total contact containment. Mention has already been made of the good results of applying pneumatic splintage as primary

treatment for fractures (see page 42). The traction effect is not present, but further shortening is prevented by the containment of the limb within a rigid cylinder preventing the outward bulge of the soft tissue, including muscles, which would need to occur for this to take place (see Fig. 5.5, page 43).

When applying these principles to arm orthoses, note that as the fractures treated are not weight bearing one of the major forces producing hydrodynamic compression and contact is absent and only the gravitational effects of the limb-part weight are available for this. The direction of this force is highly variable. In the main, therefore, in the arm the function is that of three-point fixation.

16

Knee orthoses (KO)

These are prescribed for two main groups:

1. The older patient suffering from rheumatoid or other forms of arthritis (often affecting multiple joints) with problems of hand functions, fragile skin and poor circulation. These constitute about 95 per cent of all prescriptions and a survey (Butler *et al.*, 1983) has shown that about 50 per cent are discarded within 2 weeks. This finding has implications regarding prescription criteria, degree of beneficial effects and finance. When they are maintained they are worn for all locomotor activities. Ease of application and comfort in sitting can be vital factors in acceptance.
2. The remaining 5 per cent are worn by the young athletic patient for vigorous activities only. The disability is usually confined to one joint and any ligamentous laxity will often affect rotational instability of tibia on femur as well as the valgus/varus and anteroposterior laxity present in the other group.

MECHANICAL PROBLEMS

Mechanical problems particular to KOs are as follows:

(1) *Short lever (i.e. moment) arms*—They have, therefore, little leverage advantage and the forces resisting movement or deformation are high compared with the displacing or deforming forces (see Fig. 5.13, page 48).

(2) *The point of application of the resisting forces*—This is often over soft tissue.

(3) *That of maintaining correct position vertically and rotationally*—Such orthoses not only tend to slide down the leg under the influence of gravity (the 'suspension' problem, present in this case in both stance and in-swing phase, unlike that in prosthetics) but are also influenced by centrifugal and impact forces. The problem of maintenance of alignment of anatomical and orthotic axis (if any) is considerable. In general in attempts to secure suspension, either a band is fitted in the supra-patellar region (latex covered as used in the original patellar tendon bearing below-knee prosthesis) or plastic is moulded into this region. In women use of a suspender belt may be the easiest solution.

(4) *That, particularly in rotation, of securing a fixed point of reaction to a theoretical action*—Analysis of so-called 'de-rotational' orthoses, i.e. those that will

correct a rotational instability when it occurs, commonly suggests that they are primarily anti-rotational. Whilst they may have some secondary de-rotational activity consequent upon the elastic band used for this function, the curved contour of the band has nothing to do with rotation as is claimed.

(5) *Additionally in those orthoses that require casting* many of the patients have weak musculature and loose folds of skin, and the shape of the limb may be very different in the upright position from the lying. If possible, casting should be done with the patient standing. It may be necessary to apply a crêpe bandage or tubular elasticized stockinette to obtain a reasonable shape and the patient should be instructed then to apply a similar compression before putting the orthosis on.

TREATMENT OBJECTIVES

Treatment objectives are:

1. Rest in a position as near to full extension as possible.
2. Stabilization of the knee.
3. Control of normal or abnormal joint range.
4. Retention of heat.
5. Comfort of compression.

Rest in a chosen position as near to full extension as possible

Whilst the most efficient way to do this is a KAFO, a long leg cylinder may be prescribed in an attempt to diminish the orthotic burden in the older, frail polyarthritic patient. It can be made in a variety of materials but the heavier block leather has now been substantially replaced by plastic which can be of one piece with a longitudinal opening of various widths or in two overlapping segments. A wide opening allows the limb to be put in relatively easily but diminishes the restraint provided, particularly where there is some fixed deformity and support is necessary. The amount of restraint may be increased by making the orthosis three-quarters encircling with a soft pull-down knee cap, threaded through D rings, with a broad padded Velcro strap at the top and bottom. The almost circumferential cylinder is much stronger but many patients find it impossible to open sufficiently and become dependent on outside help. One solution is two overlapping segments. The finished orthosis should be extended as high up the leg as is practical to maximize the length of the lever arms. Edges should always be slightly flared out to prevent a cutting edge being formed on the soft tissue of the posterior thigh.

Stabilization of the knee

Instability can be of two important different types:

1. Ligamentous laxity.
2. Joint axis change by loss of meniscus and articular cartilage or by collapse of osteoporotic bone (see Fig. 15.8, page 162).

Ligamentous laxity

This will be correctable in recumbency but recurs on weight bearing. Provided only one major ligament is lax it is more easy to stabilize than (2) for reasons already given. Both can be corrected in recumbency but occur on weight bearing and during walking; may be significantly affected by disease of other joints above and below the knee. If there is a general ligamentous laxity then three-point fixation is not available, and a greater number of forces must be used and a very efficient orthosis is required if it is to work at all. With bony changes three-point fixation may still be possible if the appropriate ligament is of normal length, but the limb may need to be held in over-correction. These factors may be assessed clinically and radiologically and must be assessed before considering whether a KO can be of use or whether a KAFO is required.

Joint axis change

This may be correctable and in this case stabilization should be the orthotic aim; if not, then support will be required.

During walking the situation may be significantly affected in both types by disease of other joints above and below the knee.

Depending on the degree of the problem various levels of orthotic efficiency can be used apart from the long cylinder. A skeletal version of this is the supracondylar knee orthosis (Fig. 16.1(a)). This uses three-point fixation and as illustrated does this in one plane only; deformation occuring in more than one plane will need appropriate placement of the pressure areas which are predetermined clinically. Such a device is light for its strength but has problems of assumption requiring a very mobile, slim foot and ankle. To overcome such difficulties divided plastic cuffs with anterior or posterior openings are joined with knee hinges which may be free or lockable, and this allows more comfortable sitting (Fig. 16.1(b)). Where the cuffs are under considerable mechanical stress, if they are to retain their original fit and their efficiency, closure must include the interlocking tongue and slot method used for quadrilateral sockets (see Fig. 5.7(b), page 44). This can pose a problem for patients with poor hand function.

To overcome the axis alignment problem and to control slight valgus or varus deformity in patients with only slight or no swelling, the TVS (telescopic valgus/varus support) or CARS-UBC (Canadian Arthritis and Rheumatism Society, University of British Columbia) brace was developed (Cousins *et al.*, 1977) (Fig. 16.2). It is supplied complete with a comprehensive leaflet giving contra-indications (for example, a flexion deformity of greater than 15 degrees) but requires expert fitting and special training of the patient in the correct application. Although this is simple physically, many patients are confused, even when the upper end is labelled (as it should always be); some never achieve assumption even after repeated instruction. It is advisable to determine their potential in this respect at an early stage. Again the brace applies contact only at the areas of three-point pressure. Two of these are plastic and joined by the telescopic bar to allow knee flexion and also by a flexible nylon rod which as it bends keeps these pads in correct alignment with the leg. The third point is a leather pad which does not move on flexion. Where there is

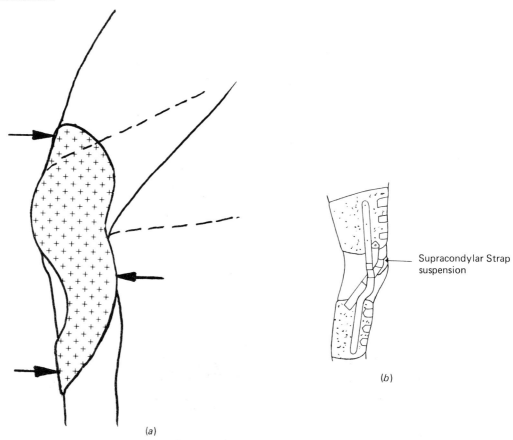

Fig. 16.1 (a) Skeletal version of the supracondylar knee orthosis. It is of particular value in preventing hyperextension but on sitting there is an awkward projection. (b) Divided plastic cuffs with a supracondylar strap suspension.

swelling with muscle wastage the bar and rod will contact the knee. To some limited extent this can be overcome by lifting the pads away from the leg by insertion of dense foam beneath the pressure pads. A waist belt may be needed for suspension. It has therefore a useful function in a limited number of carefully selected patients.

Transient joint axis change

Instability may occur transiently, often unpredictably and usually under considerable mechanical stress, as in sport. This may include the fore and aft laxity of cruciate ligament injuries or, in multiple ligamentous injuries, the so-called 'lateral pivot', an abnormal horizontal rotation of the medial tibial condyle about a longitudinal axis in the anterior part of the lateral compartment (Fig. 16.3).

The only type of orthosis that can possibly match the high level of mecha-

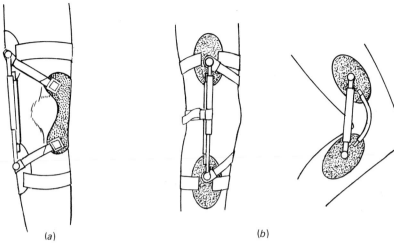

Fig. 16.2 Modification of the CARS–UBC knee brace. (a) Anterior with knee extended. (b) Relative change of length of segments (nylon bar anteriorly and telescopic bar posteriorly) on flexion, seen from lateral view.

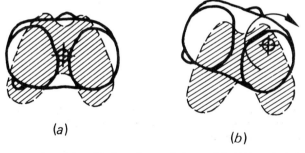

Fig. 16.3 Rotational instability of the knee, the so-called pivot shift. (a) Normal relationship of the femur (shaded) to the upper surface of the tibia looking downwards. The rotation that occurs does so about the axis marked in the region of the tibial spine. (b) Owing to ligamentous damage the axis has shifted as indicated and the tibia can now rotate abnormally on the femur as shown.

nical stresses needs to have a strong rigid frame as a basis for the mounting of various straps. A typical design is the Lennox–Hill Brace (Kennedy and Fowler, 1971; Nicholas, 1973; Hanswyk and Baker, 1982) (Fig. 16.4). The frame is of metal and has hinges. It has a rear opening and is maintained on the limb by posterior elastic bands crossed or parallel depending on patient preference. Suspension depends partly on the frame being made to a plaster cast, and therefore perfectly contoured, and on reinforcement by a suprapatellar band.

As the brace has many potential functions the other parts are added according to the requirements, e.g. it can provide pads to apply three-point fixation or bands to resist tibial displacement. The anteroposterior resisting strap passes across the tibial tubercle.

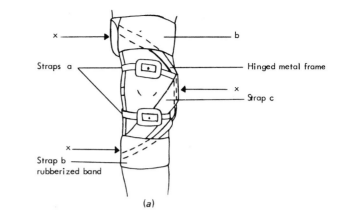

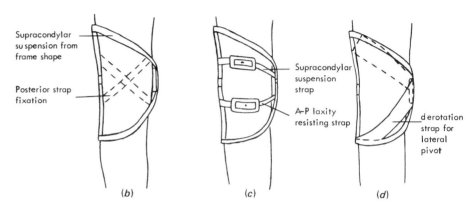

Fig. 16.4 Lennox–Hill brace. (a) Total components. xxx = Three-point fixation. (b), (c) and (d) are various components of the brace.

Pivotting is resisted by a strong longitudinal elastic strap applied next to the skin which encircles the knee in a spiral underneath all other parts. Should any pivotting occur energy is loaded into this band, and the stored energy released as the stress diminishes, reducing the displacement.

To aid in the prevention of longitudinal rotation on knee flexion and to assist suspension two further elastic straps are provided, one at each end of the frame, which are circumferential. This rather complex device requires a clear understanding of the function by the prescriber and orthotist and a user with normal hands and agile mind. It has a limited but vital role in some vigorous sporting activities such as skiing and in American football where it may have opened up a new orthotic dimension as a blunt aggressive weapon which could cause it to be banned in many circumstances. It is also used post-operatively as a protective device. This particular brace can only be obtained by sending a cast to the USA and is covered by patents, but similar devices are gradually becoming directly available in the UK, e.g. the CAM-AM brace.

Control of normal, abnormal joint range

As is so often the case overlapping of function occurs and to some extent this comes within resting and stabilizing categories. A specific single-function orthosis of this class is the Swedish brace (Lehneis, 1968; Farncombe, 1980) for the restriction of hyperextension (Fig. 16.5). This is used in rheumatoid and stroke patients. It consists of a plastic-coated aluminium frame with webbing straps across the top and bottom anteriorly and a padded band across the popliteal fossa. The upright bars are optimally pre-flexed to improve sitting cosmesis. It is front opening, the straps are easily secured, it is light and has a supracondylar suspension. Because there are no articulations there are no alignment problems and its constraints on other movements are modest.

If limitation of extension is required appropriate stops can be inserted into the hinges of the orthoses with plastic cuffs.

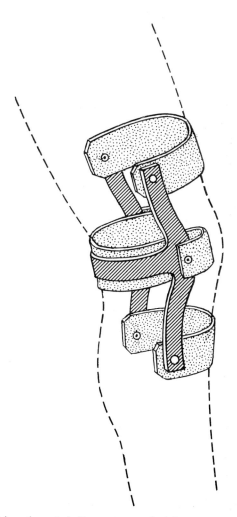

Fig. 16.5 Swedish brace for control of hyperextension. Shaded areas represent metal, dots soft straps.

The commonest orthosis used at the knee level is some form of elasticated circumferential orthosis, the simplest of which is the crêpe bandage which can be very successful provided that the bandage is of a type that retains its elasticity for a reasonable period; unfortunately, these are now relatively rare. An advantage is that it can be adjusted individually by the patient. Preformed tubular elastic examples of varying strength and design have the disadvantage of having to be worked over the foot and up the leg. A variant is to provide a longitudinal opening so that the splint can be wrapped around the knee and closed either with straps and buckles or with touch and hold. Much will then depend on the patient's hand capacity both to manipulate the fastenings and to apply adequate tension to the bands.

Elasticized stockinette can be obtained which exerts a constant pressure unrelated to the variations in diameter and can be adjusted by the patient by doubling or trebling the thickness. As this can be done on the leg it means that the tube can be pulled on at its weakest tension. Obviously the degree of limitation of movement is very slight and in an endeavour to 'improve' this, hinged metal side members are inserted into medial and lateral leather pockets (cinch brace*) (Butler *et al.*, 1983).

As in any mechanical system the weakest part yields first and under stress the stretching of the elastic negates any effect the side members might have. This was tested experimentally by inserting hinged rubber side members and by performing gait assessment in a well-equipped laboratory with the orthodox and modified orthosis on three patients. No objective difference in gait, ability to transfer from chair to walking or in deformity was noted. Subjectively one patient detected no difference whilst two found that the modification was a considerable improvement, the orthosis fitted more closely to the knee contour and was lighter. In another patient who simply had the side members removed no change was appreciated. The leather front panel inserted into the cinch brace and straps tend to limit flexion especially when the brace is felt lined. This gives a feeling of security, particularly in those patients who tend to walk with a straight knee in order to 'guard' it.

Retention of heat

Patients vary considerably in this respect, some finding it beneficial and others that it worsens their symptoms. A trial with a crêpe bandage is a useful guide to prescription.

Comfort of compression

This may be either local or circumferential. This function although vague in its mechanism is a pragmatic reality. The degree of comfort produced is very individual and in the swollen knee can vary during the day. Easy adjustment of tension can be a desirable attribute in circumferential orthoses.

---

* Cince is a saddle girth and to cinch is to pull in tightly. The name of this brace derives from straps at top and bottom.

All orthoses may, without any visible effect, to some extent unload over-stressed hypersensitive structures both in the undeformed and deformed, but the potentiality decreases rapidly as the deformity increases and interface discomfort increases.

17

Combined trunk and body brace (HKAFO)

Strictly this should be designated TLSHAFO but a system can become a tyr
anny and HKAFO seems to have been adopted by mutual but unorganized
consent.

USES

The use of these orthoses for congenital dislocation of the hip and for Perthes
disease has been dealt with (see page 117). The remaining uses are concerned
with neurological conditions:

1. Paraplegic from traumatic or congenital lesions of the spinal cord or high
    cauda equina. These are usually associated with sensory loss (including
    loss of joint position appreciation—proprioception) and commonly with
    urinary and faecal incontinence, and in the case of myelomeningocele
    hydrocephalus more or less controlled by a valve draining cerebrospinal
    fluid from the ventricles of the brain into the blood stream, pleura or peri-
    toneum. It can give rise to some central instability. This type is usually
    mainly flaccid.
2. Widespread flaccid paralysis without sensory loss resulting from acute
    anterior poliomyelitis.
3. Cerebral palsy of the spastic and athetoid types with sensory apprecia-
    tion.

FUNCTIONAL REQUIREMENTS

Functionally the orthoses may be required to produce:

1. Stabilization both intrinsic and extrinsic of the skeleton.
2. Control.

176

Control

Control of hip-joint movement during walking

This is needed to avoid the four problems that reduce gait efficiency:

1. Forward flexion collapse at the hips controlled by crutches (see Fig. 5.25, page 59).
2. 'Scissoring'. This can be opposed, more successfully in the flaccid than the spastic paralysis, by extending leg orthoses up on to the trunk. There is usually a hinge between the two sections which has in the past been used only for sitting, and indeed the design did not allow low friction movement during gait (see Fig. 5.23(b), page 57).
3. 'Windswept fall-out' (see Fig. 5.23(c), page 57) the adduction of one hip and abduction of the other. This position means that the body centre of mass passes beyond the support area of the adducted leg so the normal dynamic stable stability of the pathway of the centre of mass in space is lost. Extra injection of energy is required through the crutch, at each step in the case of flaccid paralysis. In spastic paralysis the condition does not alternate but the abducted leg causes relative lengthening of the limb and the centre of mass has to be raised a greater distance than normal.
4. Posterior fall-out. This is the most devastating of the three and if the patient is near to this continuously he will not have the confidence to continue walking (see Fig. 5.23(d), page 57). If the body centre of mass passes behind the support area when the swing leg is raised from the ground by pushing upwards by the crutch on the same side, the only solution is to put the leg down again in the same position. Any attempt to move the crutches backwards moves the centre of mass in the same direction and increases the extrinsic instability. The situation is controlled by limiting the flexion of the hip (see Fig. 5.25, page 59).

Damping of the random aberrant movements that occur in athetoid cerebral palsy

This comes largely within experimental orthotics and the methods used vary from the application of weights (boots, for example, with lead soles) through various and often adjustable joint constraints (elastic, springs, hydraulic damping) to complex electronic feedback systems used mainly in spastic conditions with the input derived from the angular change in joint movement translated into auditory signals to which the patient can respond more or less effectively after a prolonged period of training. This is an area in which progress can be expected as the present interest in Functional Electrical Stimulation grows.

DESIGN

The design of orthoses for paraplegia has to allow for:

1. The components of locomotion and of gait.

2. The practical problems in achieving joint control.
3. The essential criteria of locomotor independence:
   (a) Low-energy ambulation.
   (b) Independent transfer from sitting to walking.
   (c) Independent assumption and removal of the orthosis (doff and don).

EXAMPLES

Examples of these braces are:

1. The swivel walker (Rose and Henshaw, 1972, 1973).
2. The Hip Guidance Orthosis (hgo) (Rose, 1979).
3. HKAFO using either cables or a gearbox to attempt to transfer energy directly from one leg to another, an example of which is the LSU (Louisiana State University) Reciprocating Gait Orthosis.

This is an area in which all therapies—surgery, orthotics and physical—must be closely integrated. Orthotics has now assumed two hitherto neglected roles:

1. That orthotic design based on a clear understanding of the components of locomotion and gait combined with sound engineering principles dictate the pattern of other therapies. It follows that their exponents must thoroughly understand the design principles. With this knowledge surgical and physical therapy objectives become clearly defined, removing inefficient trial-and-error empiricism which has the advantage of freeing the severely handicapped for the many other tasks of living including education. This represents a reversal of roles, as traditionally orthotics has been regarded as some sort of last remedy when other therapies have reached the end of their capabilities.
2. To the traditional orthotic role of joint stabilization has been added that of control of joint movement during ambulation.

From the mechanical point of view all devices used for joint control and transmission of energy need to be rigid. Failure to attain this leads to flexing under mechanical stress which means that the limb pathway will be inaccurate and the problems of achieving joint control will still occur. Additionally, energy needed for the propulsion will be lost in flexing the frame. It is this absolute need for structural rigidity that has, to date, dictated the metal construction. A clear distinction has to be made between rigidity of structure and rigidity of control. Patients respond badly to the feeling that they are encapsulated in a walking machine which allows them no available independent control tolerance to deal with variations in surface. Variations will also inevitably come from their own modification of movement, e.g. changes in placement of crutches on successive steps or the need to go round corners. This has often been a problem in some designs when by various means one leg movement has been interconnected with the other.

The hinges themselves must be of a ball-bearing low-friction type and will contain stops to control range when walking, with releasable stops to allow sitting (Fig. 17.1).

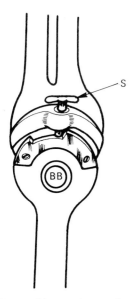

Fig. 17.1 Schematic drawing of bearing hinge used at the hip joint of a hgo. The stop (S) prevents excessive flexion. It is spring loaded and can be raised for sitting. BB = Ball bearing.

For independence of donning the most difficult problem is the insertion of orthodox spurs into the shoe tube. Poliomyelitic patients using a KAFO adopt the method of never taking them out and removing the foot from the shoe. This is aided, as is the reverse process, by unlocking the knee. This is difficult for patients with insensitive feet who do not know where their feet and toes are in space and must for this reason and for safety purposes put the boot on under complete vision. It is more difficult for them because not all devices unlock at the knee, and even with this, the hip articulation does not allow the external rotation of the hip necessary for the footwear to be brought into view and not obscured by the flexed knee. The solution to this problem is to provide a tray into which the shoe can be easily positioned and retained. This tray can be slightly curved longitudinally to facilitate walking and is fixed to the side bars in 6 degrees calcaneus deformity.

Ideally, as with all complex orthoses, a clear specification, instruction manuals and courses, and measuring charts should be available (Fig. 17.2). In the fitting stage alignment of the anatomical and orthotic joints must be precise if problems noted with mal-alignment at the knee are to be avoided. This is particularly so if the hips are not symmetrical as in dislocation of one hip, which is not a bar to usage of these orthoses.

Swivel walker (Fig. 17.3)

This allows ambulation in paraplegia up to cervical six level. It is used mainly in spina bifida and has been successfully used in age ranges from 1 to 40. It makes use of components of locomotion and components of gait.

Components of locomotion

1. Stabilization:
   (a) Intrinsic: complete exoskeleton (see Fig. 3.6, page 24), best by stabilization with fully extending joints. More than 15 degrees of flexion of the knees requires surgical straightening ideally.
   (b) Extrinsic: enlarged footplates (see Fig. 3.8, page 25).
2. Propulsion: footplate bearings placed an appropriate distance behind the body centre of mass. When the one footplate is raised from the ground by inertial forces generated by sharp lateral trunk movement, this relationship ensures that the lifted footplate rotates forward without further muscular effort. The rate at which this occurs can be enhanced by inertial input from the arms and trunk.
3. Control:
   (a) Intrinsic: feedback from the sensory/nonsensory interface.
   (b) Extrinsic: rhythmic noise from the footplate activity.

Components of gait

1. Horizontal rotation—occurs at footplate bearings.
2. Lateral rocker at footplate which has a 7 degree dihedral (Fig. 17.4).

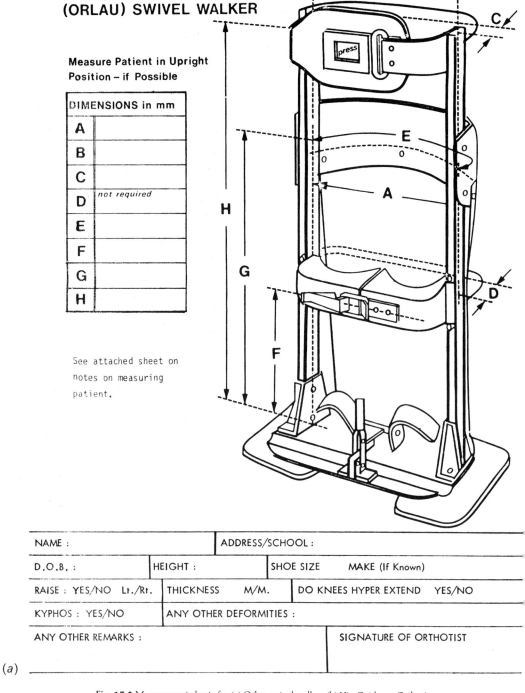

MEASUREMENT SHEET (ORLAU) SWIVEL WALKER

Measure Patient in Upright Position – if Possible

DIMENSIONS in mm	
A	
B	
C	
D	not required
E	
F	
G	
H	

See attached sheet on notes on measuring patient.

NAME :		ADDRESS/SCHOOL :	
D.O.B. :	HEIGHT :	SHOE SIZE	MAKE (If Known)
RAISE : YES/NO Lt./Rt.	THICKNESS M/M.	DO KNEES HYPER EXTEND YES/NO	
KYPHOS : YES/NO	ANY OTHER DEFORMITIES :		
ANY OTHER REMARKS :		SIGNATURE OF ORTHOTIST	

(a)

Fig. 17.2 Measurement sheets for (a) Orlau swivel walker; (b) Hip Guidance Orthosis.

MEASUREMENT SHEET
(ORLAU) HIP GUIDANCE ORTHOSIS

See attached
notes on measuring patient.

**Measure Patient in Upright
Position – if Possible**

DIMENSIONS in mm	
A	
B	
C	
D	
E	
F₁	
F₂	
G₁	
G₂	
H₁	
H₂	

This measurement sheet is not for

caliper dimensions

Calipers to be measured and supplied

by individual Orthotic Appliance

Makers.

NAME :	ADDRESS/SCHOOL :		
D.O.B. :	HEIGHT :	SHOE SIZE	MAKE (If Known)
RAISE : YES/NO Lt./Rt.	THICKNESS M/M.	DO KNEES HYPER EXTEND YES/NO	
KYPHOS : YES/NO	ANY OTHER DEFORMITIES :		
ANY OTHER REMARKS :		SIGNATURE OF ORTHOTIST	

(b)

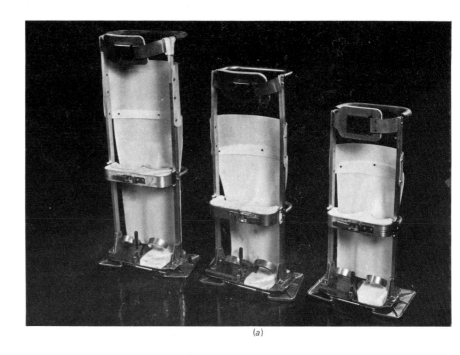

(a)

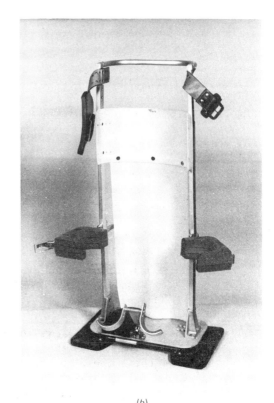

(b)

Fig. 17.3 (a) Modern Orlau swivel walkers. (b) To show front opening design.

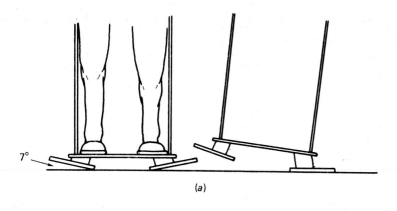

(a)

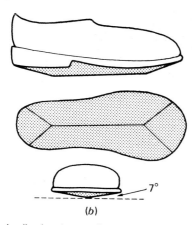

(b)

Fig. 17.4 (a) Dihedral swivel walker footplates to allow side-to-side rocking. (b) Shape of the sole of the hgo footplate for a similar purpose.

Advantages

1. Low energy required.
2. Can be used for standing at 12 months of age and walking during the next 12 months. It therefore matches the normal developmental stages and is consequently of both physical and psychological advantage. The erect position with mechanical stress through the skeleton reduces spontaneous fractures and helps with genito-urinary drainage.
3. Hands are free. This combined with the erect position may have specific advantages for some adults, e.g. those who control machines only designed for a standing operator, such as a lathe.
4. Can be used with associated hemiplegia, with a spinal orthosis, dislocated hips and up to cervical six level.
5. Modern design with the front opening allows independent doff and don.
6. Is sufficiently strong to be used with crutches in swing-through gait in older stronger patients when needed. This enables slopes of up to 1 in 20 to be negotiated, low single steps and a variety of outdoor surfaces such as turf and tarmac.

7.   Is now a modular commercial product, widely available with high reliabi-
     lity and wear characteristics.

Disadvantages

1.   Slow speed; maximum is 25 per cent normal pace.
2.   Without crutches gives level walking only.
3.   Movement pattern has only the one element of normal gait and this re-
     duces dynamic cosmesis.

In the check-out of this orthosis there are three major factors, all of which require knowledge of the position and centre of mass of the combined system of
patient and orthosis. This can be determined by a cheap, portable home-made
device consisting of a wooden platform of suitable size balanced on a knife-
edge fulcrum (also of wood) running transversely under the middle. One end
rests on a bathroom scale and a weight is placed on the platform at this end
(Fig. 17.5). The reading is noted and the patient in the orthosis is placed on the
platform and moved backwards or forwards until the reading returns to the

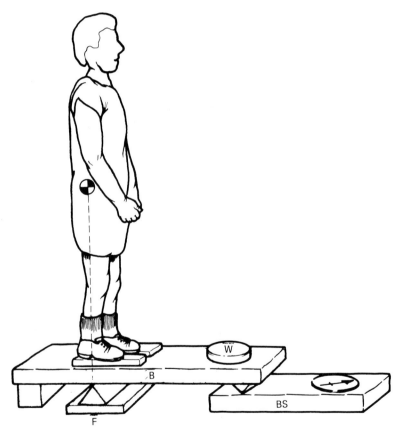

Fig. 17.5 Wooden platform B is balanced on a transverse fulcrum (F). At one end there is a knife
edge which rests on a bathroom scale (BS) and a weight (W) is put in position. When the centre
of mass of the child plus the orthosis is put over the fulcrum the reading on the bathroom scale
will return to that noted with the weight only.

previous figure. The centre of mass then lies above the fulcrum as it is only in this position that it has no effect on the balance. It is marked on the footplate. The patient is then turned sideways and the process repeated. With this information it can be ensured:

1.   That the centre of mass is in the centre of the plate in the sagittal plane thus ensuring maximum extrinsic stability.
2.   That the centre of mass is 1–2 cm ahead of the bearing axis depending on the size of the patient.
3.   That in the coronal plane the centre of mass is central between the footplates. If this is not so one footplate will easily lift from the floor and the other with difficulty or not at all. This is apt to occur if the legs or spine are deformed and if these cannot be corrected it will be necessary to reposition the footplates asymmetrical to the splint but with the mid-point under the centre of mass.

There is a need for compromise in the spacing of the footplates. The nearer together the shorter the step length but the easier to get the plates from the ground as the necessary lateral shift of the centre of mass is small. As speed is

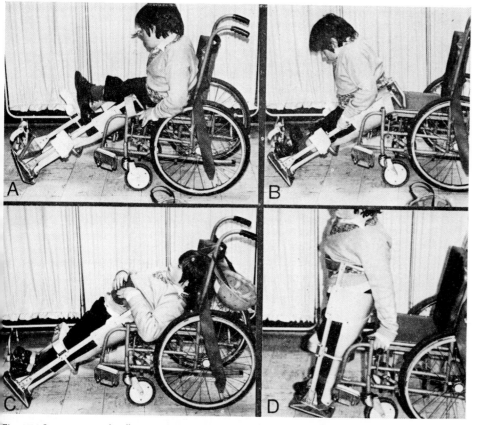

Fig. 17.6 Stages in a swivel-walker patient getting from sitting to standing. (A) Patient brings swivel walker into position as he sits on the chair and lifts legs on to the plastic trays. (B) The patient slides down into position. (C) Closing the front fastening containing components at foot, knee and chest height. (D) Elevation to standing position using the arms.

determined both by step length and cadence such a position would require very rapid repetition of steps to produce a reasonable speed. Experimentally it has been determined that one-fifth body height between bearing centres is the optimum for speed and energy consumption. Of course, in the early stages with a young child learning to walk it is helpful to move the plates closer for ease of usage and to accept lower speeds, moving to an optimum when skill and confidence are acquired. Parents and teachers asked that the design should be modified to allow sitting. This would have required the insertion of nine sets of hinges which would jeopardize essential rigidity. A technique which combined well with the independent doff and don was devised as shown in Fig. 17.6. The patient could get into the splint and walk independently in 30–60 seconds and could, of course, reverse the process.

Hip guidance orthosis (hgo) (Fig. 17.7)

Whilst swivel walkers enable walking early in life to be achieved their speed surface limitations and their somewhat penguin-like pattern of progression made the development of reciprocal orthoses with better characteristics eminently desirable. The hgo was therefore produced. It makes use of components of locomotion and components of gait.

Components of locomotion

1. Stabilization:
   (a) Intrinsic: crutches plus hip articulated KAFOs (long leg braces with or without knee articulations for sitting).
   (b) Extrinsic: crutches plus limitation of hip flexion range when walking.
2. Propulsion:
   (a) Swing: gravity causing pendulum action of the leg.
   (b) Stance: uphill by arm and trunk muscles reacting through crutches with inertial enhancement from the previous stance energy of the other leg.
   (c) Downhill: gravitational lowering of body mass.
3. Control:
   (a) Intrinsic: feedback from the sensory/non-sensory interface.
   (b) Extrinsic: hip articulation with limited flexion range.

Components of gait

1. Leg pendulum—swing.
2. Leg vaulting—stance.
3. Lateral rocker at footwear/floor level. This is an area where an attempt to imitate the normal has not proved satisfactory for a number of reasons:
   (a) That normally in mid-stance the pelvis adducts not abducts. This is to reduce the rise of the body centre of mass. An articulation that depends on abduction will cause increased energy cost and consideration has to be given to whether this can be minimized (see Fig. 6.2, page 71).

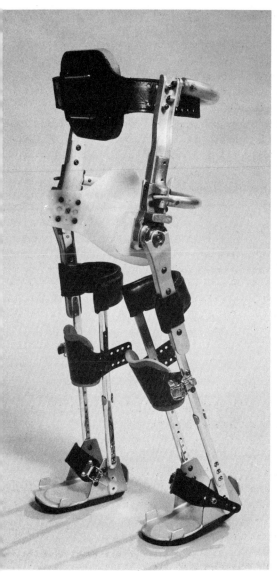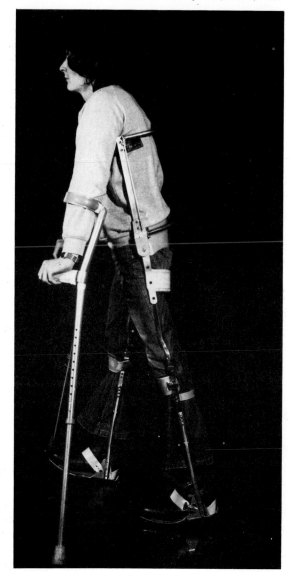

Fig. 17.7 Hip Guidance Orthosis.

(b)   That an extra joint promotes flexibility and this increases as it wears.
(c)   That the commonly used comb joint has a high friction at best and frequently binds completely.

Advantages

1.   Low energy requirements.
2.   Speed over 50 per cent normal rate of walking.
3.   Can surmount a single step of 15 cm (6 in) and a slope, up or down of one in ten.
4.   Can be used on all surfaces; for example, roads and fields.

5. Very acceptable dynamic cosmetic walking pattern.
6. Independent doff and don and transfer from sitting to walking.
7. Available for children from 4 years onwards and adults.

Disadvantages

1. Associated hemiplegia and marked spinal instability contra-indicated.
2. Crutches are needed.
3. Because of the 'hairpin' design, attainment of rigidity is a very significant engineering problem which increases with the height and weight of the patient. A mechanically more efficient structure could be achieved by the placement of a strut between the feet. Unfortunately, to do so would be to revert to swivel walking. Reciprocal gait only occurs where there is change in length between the feet. It is not possible to produce a telescopic strut that will also completely resist compression as it elongates. At present, therefore, a strong metallic structure is necessary. Functional Electrical Stimulation (FES) is possible in upper motor neurone lesions because the peripheral nerve and muscle remain functional and it is only the inability of the patient to pass a message from the brain to the nerve that causes paralysis. This has opened up possibilities of a hybrid apparatus in which at an appropriate time stimulation of the abductor muscles of the hip will reinforce the mechanical resistance to adduction. In these circumstances it will be possible to make the body segment at least in appropriately strong plastic and to make it conform to the body shape. Additional uses of FES are to activate the hip extensors to aid the 'uphill' portion of stance and to stimulate the quadriceps to aid standing. Active research in several centres has demonstrated the practicability of these concepts.

Assessment (including energy consumption) of the results of the usage of hgo and swivel walkers of modern design in the first 100 cases showed a substantial improvement over other reported types used for lesions at similar levels; and showed the practicability of orthoses at higher levels than previously used.

HKAFO with inter-activation of leg braces (Fig. 17.8)

Early varieties of this type were reported by Scrutton in the UK and McLaurin in Canada (Motlock, 1976). In the former the legs were interconnected by two Bowden cables attached to outriggers mounted at the upper end of the leg segments just below the hip hinge used during walking. This means that as one leg flexes the other must extend, and intrinsic stability is achieved because both hips cannot flex simultaneously. Equally, of course, they cannot extend together but this is not a problem in any device as the natural restraint of the anatomical hip protects the orthosis from excessive movement.

Theoretically, therefore, the swinging forward of the one leg under the influence of gravity assists the other in the 'uphill' phase of stance, and in the 'downhill' phase the flexion of the other leg is assisted. In practice some energy must be lost in the friction of the cables. McLaurin's gearbox reduced this and it could also be put into 'neutral' to allow sitting. The chief disadvantage, and it is a serious one, is the rigidity of control that such systems impose. The 'LSU Reciprocating Gait Orthosis' also uses this system. It consists of conforming plastic KAFOs specially reinforced at the ankle to maintain a rigid right angle. These are joined through hinges at the hip level to metal side bars connected at the nipple line by a covered metal spacer bar at the back and a soft band anteriorly; and at the pelvic level by a narrow metal band enshrouded in a broad plastic band moulded to a cast of the body. Very complete details of manufacture from a standard range of centrally manufactured modular parts with fitting instructions are available. In 1983 it was reported that 95 cases of spina bifida, 18 of traumatic paraplegia, 15 of muscular dystrophy, 8 of cerebral palsy, 1 of multiple sclerosis and 1 of sacral agenesis had been supplied with this type of orthosis (McCall *et al.*, 1983; Douglas *et al.*, 1983).

The clinical findings of the 22 myelomeningocele cases reported in some detail do not enable direct comparison to be made with other types from the point of view of efficiency of walking nor are details available of transfer, or of independent doff and don. Some cases have asymmetrical lesions and theoretically this means that muscle power from one leg can be used in the other, but it is not yet clear whether this outweighs the problems of control.

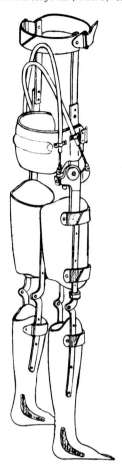

Fig. 17.8 LSU reciprocating gait orthosis.

Bibliography and further reading

BIBLIOGRAPHY

Abbott, E. G. (1911). Simple, rapid and complete reduction of deformity in fixed lateral curvature of the spine. *NY Med. J.* **93**, 1217–19.

Ahlgren, S. A. and Hansen, T. (1978). The use of lumbo-sacral corsets prescribed for low back pain. *Prosth. Orth. Int.* **2**, 101–4.

Aitken, D. M. (1928). Curvature of the spine. In *The Robert Jones Birthday Volume*, p. 243. Oxford: Oxford Medical Publications.

Appleton, A. B. (1934). Postural deformities and bone growth. *Lancet* **i**, 451.

Bainbridge, S. (1979). *National Health Surgical Footwear—A Study of Patient Satisfaction*. London: HMSO.

Barnes, G. H. (1970). Skin health and stump hygiene. In *Artificial Limbs*, p. 114. New York: Robert E. Krieger.

Bisgrove, J. G. (1964). A new functional dynamic wrist extension—finger flexion hand splint. *Arch. Phys. Med. Rehab.* **8**, 162.

Blount, W. P. and Moe, J. H. (1973). *The Milwaukee Brace*. Baltimore: Williams & Wilkins.

Bobechko, W. P., McLaurin, C. A. and Motlock, W. M. (1968). Toronto orthosis for Legg Perthes' disease. *Artif. Limbs* **12**, 36.

BRADU (Biomechanical Research and Development Unit, DHSS) Report (1979). Dewar, M. and Wilde, G. Weight bearing characteristics of the Stanmore Caliper, p. 234.

Brandt, P. W. (1982). The insensitive foot (including leprosy). In *Disorders of the Foot*, Ed. M. Jahss, p. 1266. Philadelphia: W. B. Saunders.

Brotherton, B. J. and McKibben B. (1977). Perthes' disease treated by prolonged recumbency and femoral head containment. A long term approach. *J. Bone Jnt. Surg.* **59B**, 8.

Butler, P. B., Evans, G. A., Rose, G. K. and Patrick, J. H. (1983). A review of selected knee orthoses. *Br. J. Rheumatol.* **22**, 109.

Catachis, C. S. (1973). Cervical spine motion in normal women—radiographic study of effect of cervical collars. *Arch. Phys. Med. Rehabil.* **54**, 161.

Catteral, A. (1971). The natural history of Perthes' disease. *J. Bone Jnt. Surg.* **53B**, 37.

Charnley, J. (1950). *The Mechanics of Fracture Treatment. Modern Trends in Orthopaedics*, Vol. **23**, Ed. H. Platt, Chapter II. London: Butterworths.

Cousins, S. J., Lusby, D. L. V. and Chodera, J. (1977). Assessment and field trial of the Canadian Arthritis and Rheumatism Society–University of British Columbia orthosis for valgus/varus knee instability (CARS–UBC brace). *Annual Report of the Biomechanical Research and Development Unit*, Roehampton.

Craig, J. J. and van Vuren, J. (1976). The importance of gastrocnemius recession in the correction of equinus deformity in cerebral palsy. *J. Bone Jnt. Surg.* **58B**, 84.

Curtis, B. H., Gunther, S. F., Gossling, M. R. and Paul, S. W. (1974). Treatment of Legg Perthes' disease with a Newington Ambulatory abduction brace. *J. Bone Jnt. Surg.* **56B**, 1135.

Davies, F. J., Fry, L. R., Lippert, F. G., Simons, B. C. and Remington, J. (1974). The patellar tendon bearing brace: report on 16 patients. *J. Trauma* **14**, 216.

Davies, P. R. (1956). Variations of human intra-abdominal pressure during weight lifting in different postures. *J. Anat.* **90**, 601.

Davies, P. R. (1959). Posture of the trunk during lifting of weights. *Br. Med. J.* **i**, 87.

Davies, P. R. and Troup, J. D. G. (1964). Pressures in the trunk cavities when pulling, pushing and lifting. *Ergonomics* **7**, 465–74.

Deane, G. and Grew, N.D. (1978). Some physical effects on lumbar support orthoses. In *Orthopaedic Engineering* 39, Eds D. Harris and K. Copeland. London: Biological Engineering Soc.

Dempster, W. T. (1961). Free Body Diagrams as an approach to the mechanics of human posture and locomotion. In *Biomechanical Studies of the Musculo-Skeletal System*, Ed. F. G. Evans. Springfield, Ill.: Charles C. Thomas.

Dixon, A. St. J., Owen Smith, B. D. and Harrison, R. A. (1972). Cold sensitive non-specific low back pain. *Chem. Trades J.* **9 (4)**, 16.

Douglas, R., Lavson, P. F., D'Ambrosia, R. and McCall, R. S. (1983). The LSU reciprocation–gait orthosis. *Orthopaedics* **6 (7)**, 834.

Dounis, E., Steventon, R. D. and Wilson, R. S. E. (1980). The use of a portable oxygen consumption meter (Oxylog) for assessing efficiency of crutch walking. *J. Med. Eng. Technol.* **4 (6)**, 296.

Evans, D. L. and Lloyd Roberts, G. C. (1958). Treatment of Legg–Calve–Perthes' disease. A comparison of in-patient and out-patient methods. *J. Bone Jnt. Surg.* **40B**, 182.

Farncombe, P. M. (1980). The Swedish knee cage—management of the hyperextended hemiplegic knee. *Physiotherapy* **66**, 33.

Fishman, S., et al. (1982). *Metabolic Measures in the Evaluation of Prosthetic and Orthotic Devices.* Research Division, College of Engineering Report. New York University.

Frankel, V. H. and Burnstein, A. H. (1970). *Orthopaedic Biomechanics.* Philadelphia: Lea and Febiger.

Frejka, B. (1941). Praventation der angerborenam Huftgelensluxation durch das Abduktionspolster. *Wien. Med. Wochenschr.* **91**, 523.

Frost, H. M. (1973). *Orthopaedic Biomechanics.* Springfield, Ill.: Charles C. Thomas.

Fulford, G. E. (1978). The problems associated with flail feet in children and their treatment with orthoses. *J. Bone Jnt. Surg.* **60B**, 93–5.

Hall, J. E. and Miller, W. (1963). Prefabrication of Milwaukee braces. *J. Bone Jnt. Surg.* **56A**, 1963.

Hanswyk, E. P. van and Baker, B. E. (1982). Orthotic management of knee injuries in athletics with the Lennox–Hill orthosis. *Orthot. Prosthet.* **36**, 4.23.

Hardcastle, P. H., Ross, R., Hamalainen, M. and Mata, A. (1980). Catteral grouping of Perthes' disease. *J. Bone Jnt. Surg.* **62B**, 428.

Harris, H. E. (1973). A new orthotics terminology—a guide for its use for prescription and fee schedule. *Orthot. Prosthet.* **27**, 2.

Harris, R. J. and Beath, T. (1947). *Army Foot Survey—An Investigation of Foot Ailments in Canadian Soldiers.* Ottawa: National Research Council of Canada.

Harris, R. J. and Beath, T. (1948). Hypermobile flat-foot with short Tendo Achilles. *J. Bone Jnt. Surg.* **30A**, 116.

Harrison, M. H. M., Turner, M. H. and Nicholson, F. J. (1969). Coxa plana: results of a new form of splinting. *J. Bone Jnt. Surg.* **51A**, 1057–69.

Heize, D. (1967). Bracing design for knee joint instability. In *Principles of Lower Extremity Bracing*, Eds J. Perry and H. Hislop, pp. 92–96. American Physical Therapy Association.

Helfet, A. J. (1956). A new way of treating flat feet in children. *Lancet* **i**, 262.

Hicks, J. H. (1960). External splintage as a cause of movement. *Lancet* **ii**, 272.

James, C. C. M. and Lassman, L. P. (1972). *Spinal Dysraphism.* London: Butterworths.

James, J. I. P. (1959). Scoliosis: curve patterns. *J. Bone Jnt. Surg.* **41B**, 219.

James, J. I. P. (1960). Paralytic scoliosis: prognosis and associated muscle paralysis. *J. Bone Jnt. Surg.* **42A**, 883.

Johnson, J. T. H. and Kendall, H. O. (1964a). Isolated paralysis of serratus anterior muscle. *Orthop. Prosthet. Appl. J.* **18**, 201.

Johnson, J. T. H. and Kendall, H. O. (1964b). Isolated paralysis of serratus anterior muscle. *Orthop. Prosthet. Appl. J.* **19**, 135.

Johnson, R. M., Hart, D. L., Simmons, E. F., Ramsby, G. R. and Southwick, W. O. (1977). Cervical orthoses—a study comparing their effectiveness in restricting cervical motion in normal subjects. *J. Bone Jnt. Surg.* **59A**, 332.

Johnson, R. M., Hart, D. L. and Owen, J. R. (1978). The Yale cervical orthosis—an evaluation of its effectiveness in restricting cervical motion in normal subjects and its comparison with other cervical orthoses. *Phys. Ther.* **58**, 865.

Johnson, R. M., Owen, J. R., Hart, D. L. and Callahan, R. A. (1981). Cervical orthoses. A guide to their selection and use. *Clin. Orthop. Rel. Res.* **154**, 34.

Kennedy, J. C. and Fowler, P. J. (1971). Medial and anterior instability of the knee. *J. Bone Jnt. Surg.* **53A**, 1257.

Kennedy, J. M. (1974). *Orthopaedic Splints and Appliances.* London: Baillière Tindall.

Kite, J. H. (1963). Some suggestions on the treatment of club foot by casts. A.A.O.S. Instructional Course Lecture. *J. Bone Jnt. Surg.* **45A**, 406.

Lehmann, J. F., Delateur, B. J., Warren, C. G. and Simons, B. C. (1970a). Trends in lower extremity bracing. *Arch. Phys. Med. Rehab.* **51**, 338.

Lehmann, J. F., Warren, C. G., Delateur, B. J., Simons, B. C. and Kirkpatrick, G. S. (1970b). Biomechanical evaluation of axial loading in ischial weight bearing braces of various design. *Arch. Phys. Med. Rehab.* **51**, 331.

Lehmann, J. F., Warren, C. G., Pemberton, D. R., Simons, B. C. and Delateur, B. J. (1971). Load bearing function of patellar tendon bearing braces of various designs. *Arch. Phys. Med. Rehab.* **52**, 367.

Lehmann, J. F. and Warren, C. G. (1973). Ischial and patellar tendon weight-bearing braces: function, design, adjustment and training. *Bull. Prosthet. Res.* **10–19**, 6.

Lehmann, J. F. and Warren, C. G. (1976). Restraining force in various designs of knee ankle orthoses—Their placement and effect on the anatomical knee joint. *Arch. Phys. Med. Rehab.* **57**, 430.

Lehmann, J. F., Warren, C. G., Hertling, D., McGee, M., Simons, B. C. and Dralle, A. (1976). Craig–Scott orthosis: a biomechanical and functional evaluation. *Arch. Phys. Med. Rehab.* **57**, 438.

Lehmann, J. F. (1979). Biomechanics of ankle foot orthosis. *Arch. Phys. Med. Rehab.* **60**, 200.

Lehneis, H. R. (1968). The Swedish knee cage. *Artif. Limbs* **12**, 54.

Lovell, W. W., Hopper, W. C. and Purvis, J. M. (1978). The Scottish Rite hospital orthosis for Legg–Perthes' disease. Scientific Exhibit, Scottish Medical Association meeting, Atlanta.

McCall, R. E., Douglas, R. and Righters, N. (1983). Reciprocal gait orthosis. Its use in neurologic deficient patients. *Orthop. Trans.* **7**, 565.

McKenzie, M. W. and Buck, G. L. (1978). Combined motor and peripheral sensory insufficiency, III. Management of spinal cord injury. *Phys. Ther.* **58**, 294.

McKibben, B. (1971). Conservative management of paralytic dislocation of the hip in meningomyelocele. *J. Bone Jnt. Surg.* **53B**, 758.

Meggitt, B. F., Juett, D. A. and Smith, J. D. (1980). Cast brace function and femoral fracture repair: A biomechanical study and clinical application. *J. Bone Jnt. Surg.* **57B**, 393.

Miller, B., Dabrowski, S., Parks, B., Cassetta, M. and Watts, G. H. (1976). *Workshop Manual.* Boston: Children's Hospital Medical Center.

Morton, J. D. (1935). *The Human Foot. Its Evolution, Physiology and Functional Disorders*. New York: Columbia University Press.

Motlock, W. M. (1976). Device design in spina bifida. In *The Advances in Orthotics*, Ed. G. Murdoch, p. 415. London: Edward Arnold.

Mubarak, S., Garfin, S., Vance, R., McKinnon, B. and Sutherland, D. (1982). Pitfalls in the use of the Pavlik Harness for treatment of congenital. *J. Bone Jnt. Surg.* **63A**, 1239.

Nicholas, J. A. (1973). Reconstruction for anteromedial instability of knee. *J. Bone Jnt. Surg.* **55A**, 899.

Nichols, P. J. R., Peach, S. L., Haworth, R. J. and Ennis, J. (1978). The value of flexor huge hand splints. *Prosth. Orth. Int.* **2**, 86–94.

Norton, P. and Brown, T. (1957). The immobilisation efficiency of back braces—the effect on posture and motion of the lumbosacral spine. *J. Bone Jnt. Surg.* **39A**, 111.

Platts, R. G., Field, A. and Knight, S. (1979). Orthoses to fit shoes. *Prosth. Orth. Internat.* **3**, 89.

Ponseti, I. V. and Friedman, B. (1950). Prognosis in idiopathic scoliosis. *J. Bone Jnt. Surg.* **32A**, 381.

Ralston, A. J. and Libet, B. (1953). The question of tonus in skeletal muscle. *Am. J. Phys. Med.* **32**, 85.

Ralston, A. J. (1965). Effects of immobilisation of various body segments on the energy loss of human locomotion. *Ergonomics,* Suppl. **53**.

Ramsey, P. L., Lasser, L. and McEwen, G. D. (1976). CDH—the use of the Pavlik harness in the first six months of life. *J. Bone Jnt. Surg.* **58A**, 1000.

Raney, F. L. (1969). The Royalite Flexion Jacket in Spinal Orthotics. Committee on Prosthetic Research and Development of the National Research Council (March).

Rose, G. K. (1955). The painful heel. *Br. Med. J.* **i**, 831.

Rose, G. K. (1958). Correction of the pronated foot. *J. Bone Jnt. Surg.* **40B**, 674.

Rose, G. K. (1962). Correction of the pronated foot. *J. Bone Jnt. Surg.* **44B**, 642.

Rose, G. K. (1965). *Human Posture: Physical Medicine in Paediatrics.* London: Butterworth.

Rose, G. K. and Henshaw, J. T. (1972). A swivel walker for paraplegics; medical and technical considerations. *Biomed. Eng.* **7**, 420.

Rose, G. K. and Henshaw, J. T. (1973). Swivel walkers for paraplegics: consideration and problems in their design and application. *Bull. Prosthet. Res.* 10–20, 62–74.

Rose, G. K. (1977). Total functional assessment of orthoses. *Physiotherapy* **63**, 78.

Rose, G. K. (1979). Principles and practice of the hip guidance orthoses. *Prosth. Orth. Int.* **3**, 37.

Rose, G. K. (1980a). Orthoses for the severely handicapped—rational or empirical choice. *Physiotherapy* **66**, 76.

Rose, G. K. (1980b). Principles of splints and orthotics. In *Scientific Foundations of Orthopaedics and Traumatology*, Eds Owen, Goodfellow and Bullough, p. 443. London: William Heinemann Medical Books.

Rose, G. K. (1982). Pes planus. In *Disorders of the Foot*, Ed. M. H. Jahss, p. 486. Philadelphia: W. B. Saunders.

Rose, G. K. (1983). Orthotics. In *Clinical Orthopaedics*, Ed. N. Harris, p. 979. Bristol: Wright.

Rubin, G., Greenbaum, W. and Molack, D. (1972). A lumbo-sacral orthosis. *Bull. Prosthet. Res.* **68**, 10.

Russek, A. S. and Marks, M. (1953). Scapular fixation by bracing in serratus anterior palsy. *Arch. Phys. Med. Rehab.* **344**, 633.

Sarmiento, A. and Latta, L. L. (1981). *Closed Functional Treatment of Fractures.* Berlin: Springer-Verlag.

Schottstaedt, E. R. and Robinson, G. B. (1956). Functional bracing of the arm. *J. Bone Jnt. Surg.* **38A**, 477.

Scott, B. A. (1980). Engineering principles and fabrication techniques for the Scott-Craig long leg brace for paraplegics, selected reading. In *A review of Orthotics and Paraplegics*, Eds B. A. Mastro and R. T. Mastro, p. 281. Washington DC: The American Orthotic and Prosthetic Association.

Sheldon, W. H., Stevens, S. S. and Tucker, W. B. (1940). *The Varieties of Human Physique*. New York: Harper.

Sheldon, W. H. (1954). *Atlas of Man*. New York: Harper.

Smith, E. M. and Juvinall, R. C. (1963). Theory of feeder mechanics. *Am. J. Phys. Med.* **42**, 3.

Snyder, C. H. (1947). A sling for use in Legg–Perthes' disease. *J. Bone Jnt. Surg.* **29**, 524.

Stallard, J., Rose, G. K. and Farmer, I. R. (1978a). The ORLAU swivel walker. *Prosth. Orth. Int.* **2**, 35.

Stallard, J., Sanwarankutty, M. and Rose, G. K. (1978b). A comparison of axillary, elbow and Canadian crutches. *Rheumatol. Rehabil.* **17**, 237.

Stern, P. H., Vitarius, G. and Quint, J. (1982). Wheelchair based upper limb orthotics. *Orthot. Prosthet.* **36**, 1, 41.

Tanner, J. M. (1964). *The Physique of the Olympic Athlete*. London: George Allen & Unwin.

Tanner, J. M., Whitehouse, R. H. and Takaishi, M. (1966). Standards from birth to maturity for height–weight, height–velocity and weight–velocity. British Children 1965 Parts I & E. *Arch. Dis. Child.* **41**, 454, 613.

Trulong, X. I. and Rippel, D. V. (1979). Orthotic devices for serratus anterior palsy; some biomechanical considerations. *Arch. Phys. Med. Rehab.* **60**, 66.

Tuck, W. H. (1974). The Stanmore cosmetic caliper. *J. Bone Jnt. Surg.* **56B**, 115.

von Rosen, S. (1956). Early diagnosis and treatment of congenital dislocation of the hip joint. *Acta Orthop. Scand.* **26**, 136.

Watanabe, H., Ogata, K., Okabe, T. and Amano, T. (1978). Hand orthoses for various finger impairments; the K.U. finger splint. *Prosth. Orth. Int.* **2**, 95–100.

Waters, R. L. and Morris, J. M. (1970). Effect of spinal support on muscles of trunk. *J. Bone Jnt. Surg.* **532A**, 51.

Watts, H. G., Hall, J. E. and Stanish, W. (1977). Boston Brace system for the treatment of low thoracic lumbar scoliosis by use of a girdle without superstructure. *Clin. Orth.* **126**, 87.

Watts, H. G., Miller, B., Dabrowski, R. P. T., Parks, R. N. and Cassella, M. (1979). *Workshop Manual on Boston Brace*. Boston: Children's Hospital Medical Center.

Whitman, R. (1888). Observations of forty-five cases of flat-foot with particular reference to etiology and treatment. *Boston Med. Surg. J.* **118**, 598.

Wilkinson, J. A. (1962). Femoral anteversion in the rabbit. *J. Bone Jnt. Surg.* **44B**, 386.

Yates, G. (1976). A modular system of exoskeleton bracing. In *The Advance in Orthotics*, Ed. G. Murdoch, p. 211. London: Edward Arnold.

Zeleznik, R., Chaplin, W., Hart, D. L., Smith, H., Southwick, W. A. and Zito, M. (1978). Yale cervical orthosis. *Physio-Therapy*, **58**, 661.

FURTHER READING

Anderson, M. H. (1965). *Upper Extremity Orthotics*. Springfield, Ill.: Charles C. Thomas.

Atlas of Orthotics (1975). *Biomechanical Principles and Application*. American Academy of Orthopaedic Surgeons. St. Louis: C. V. Mosby.

Cochran, G. Van B. (1982). *A Primer of Orthopaedic Biomechanics*. Edinburgh: Churchill-Livingstone.

Frankel, V. H. and Burstein, A. H. (1970). *Orthopaedic Biomechanics*. Philadelphia: Lea and Febiger.

Frost, H. M. (1973). *Orthopaedic Biomechanics*. Springfield, Ill.: Charles C. Thomas.

Inman, V. T., Ralston, H. J. and Todd, F. (1981). *Human Walking*. Baltimore: Williams & Wilkins.

Redford, J. B. (Ed.) (1980). *Orthotics Etcetera*. Baltimore: Williams & Wilkins.

Williams, N. and Lissner, H. R. (1977). *Biomechanics of Human Movement*. Philadelphia: W. B. Saunders.

Appendix A: Materials and structures

An orthosis which has a mechanical function is a structure, one definition of which is any assemblage of materials that is intended to sustain loads. In doing this it will transmit forces, intermittently or continuously, and on occasions store energy and is, therefore, submitted to potentially destructive stresses and strains which must be resisted if it is to remain effective (see page 11).

Design of structures is an art with a scientific basis and is always a compromise between choice of materials related to the ways in which these are made into the structure. This means that there is rarely a single ideal solution. Many combinations may need to be tried before the optimum (and it is always the optimum for a particular patient) is achieved. The shortest pathway to accomplish this is by knowledge of the characteristics both of materials and of structures combined with a study of usage and particularly of failures.

In all circumstances the first objective is to identify the mechanical demands placed on the orthosis in a particular treatment. However, as we shall see, this knowledge alone does not automatically lead to a satisfactory design which is related to a number of factors:

1. Functional needs: biomechanics (see page 38), descriptive (see page 68).
2. Ideal characteristics with particular reference to fail-safe (see page 73).
3. Strength which derives from:
   (a) Materials used.
   (b) Way in which these are used—shape, heat treatment, etc.
   (c) Structural characteristics.

In general the important characteristics of materials used in orthotics are:

Strength: the ability to withstand load.
Toughness: the ability to withstand shock loading without failure.
Fatigue resistance: the ability to withstand cyclic loading.
Ductility: the ability to deform permanently before fracture.
Brittleness: an inability to withstand shock loading, i.e. lack of ductility.
Elasticity: deformation which returns to normal when loading is removed.
Corrosion resistance: the ability not to be chemically degraded in the working environment.
Density: provides a comparison of the relative weights of materials.

From an engineering point of view most of these properties derive from the basic concepts of stress and strain and their relationship to each other.

STRAIN AND STRESS

Whenever a material is loaded it deforms under the influence of the applied load. Strain is a measure of this deformation and is the ratio of the change of dimension to the original overall dimension of the test piece under consideration (Fig. A.1). Deformation takes place primarily along the line of loading and is therefore classified as compressive, tensile (Fig. A.2(a)). Shear strain (Fig. A.2(b)) occurs where equal and opposite forces parallel to each other act on the specimen and produce a 'sliding' action which turns it through an angle.

The actual strain that occurs in a material is dependent not only on the magnitude of the load but also on the area of the material over which the load is applied. It is the intensity of loading, known as stress, which determines the resulting strain. Stress is the force per unit area of the plane on which loading is applied (Fig. A.3) and like strain can be compressive, tensile or shear. In bending a combination of these stresses occur. Obviously a small load applied over a large area gives less stress than a large load on the same area.

MATERIALS

These should be appropriate to the mechanical constraints and the fact that new materials have some attractive characteristics does not necessarily mean that they are suitable for a particular purpose.

Materials are selected on the basis of a specification determined by standard test procedures. The limitation of these should be appreciated. For metals they are generally related to tensile strains, whilst the metals are used generally in compression or bending which produces both compressive and tensile loads (Fig. A.3). For plastics the situation is further complicated by the fact that they are visco-elastic, which means that their physical characteristics are modified

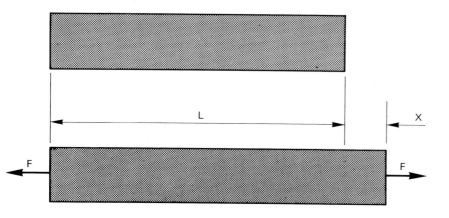

$$\text{Strain} = \frac{\text{Increase in length}}{\text{Original length}} = \frac{X}{L}$$

Fig. A.1 Definition of strain. F = Force.

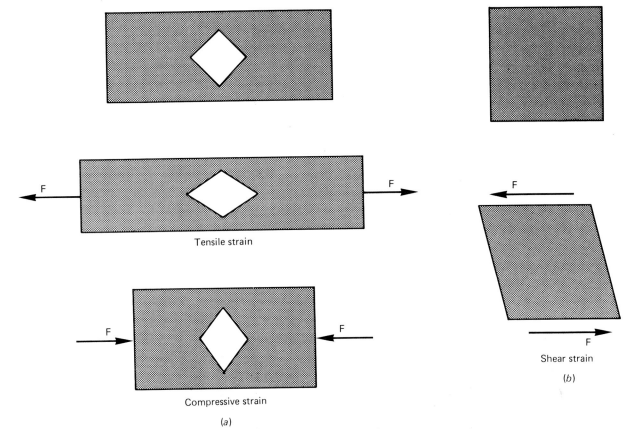

Fig. A.2 (a) Tensile and compressive strain. (b) Shear strain.

by the rate of strain applied. Whilst a vast amount of information exists, it is extremely difficult to apply this to the complex situations of an orthosis in action.

METALS

If a continuously increasing tensile force is applied to a standard specimen (a single cycle test) until it breaks and the changes that occur are measured, a stress–strain diagram will be produced (Fig. A.4) which enables various metals to be compared in relationship to design needs. Initially this will be elastic deformation, and this is temporary. If the force is discontinued then the specimen will relax to its original length, but if the force continues to rise one of two events will occur. The specimen will either suddenly fracture (brittle failure) or it will permanently deform (ductile failure) and will ultimately fracture.

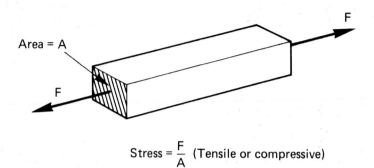

$$\text{Stress} = \frac{F}{A} \quad \text{(Tensile or compressive)}$$

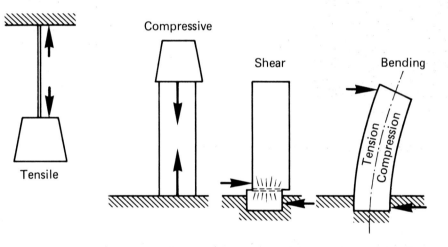

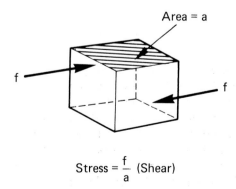

$$\text{Stress} = \frac{f}{a} \quad \text{(Shear)}$$

Fig. A.3 Definition of stress.

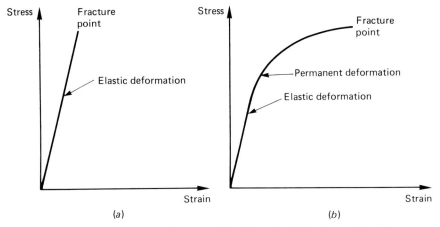

Fig. A.4 Stress–strain diagrams showing modes of failure for (a) a brittle material and (b) a ductile material.

STIFFNESS

Physical testing of practically all metals shows that equal increments of stress produce equal increments of strain within the range of loading which avoids any form of 'failure'. This means that there is a 'straight line' relationship (Fig. A.5) between stress and strain. The slope of this straight line is given by dividing the stress at any given point on the line by the strain at that same point. This slope is known as Young's modulus and is a measure of stiffness. A material that is stiff demands high stress levels to produce small amounts of strain and will have a steep slope giving a high Young's modulus, and vice versa (Fig. A.6).

Materials that behave in this proportional manner are known as elastic materials. If they are loaded within the limits of the straight line they return to their original shape and size when the load is removed.

It is important to realize that Young's modulus is *not* a measure of strength and only indicates the stiffness of a material.

STRENGTH

The strength of a material is the stress at which it fractures for a *single cycle test*. Most metals exhibit a form of failure in which increments of stress beyond a critical level produce increasing amounts of strain (Fig. A.7). The point at which that begins to happen is known as the yield point and the material is then said to undergo plastic deformation. Strain that occurs beyond the yield point is permanent and if a material was loaded, for example, to point A in Fig. A.7 it would unload along the dotted line parallel to the elastic portion of the graph. The amount of permanent deformation would be the strain at the point where the unloading line crosses the strain axis of the graph (point B). Materials that exhibit this behaviour are said to be ductile.

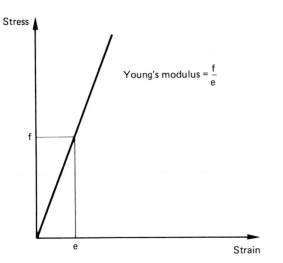

Fig. A.5 Material stiffness (Young's modulus).

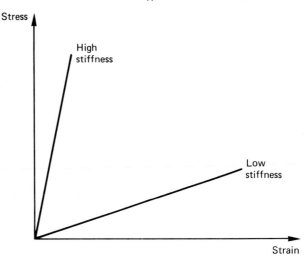

Fig. A.6 Comparison of different Young's moduli.

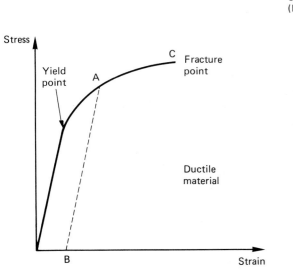

Fig. A.7 Ductile behaviour in materials.

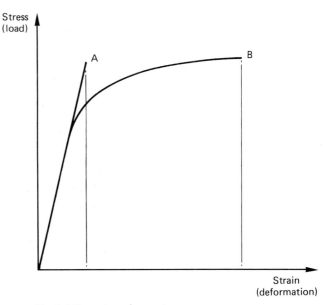

Fig. A.8 Comparison of energy to fracture.

Clearly with such a material failure begins to occur at the yield point, but is not complete until fracture occurs, at point C. The strength is the stress at that point. The increasing amounts of strain after the yield point give warning that overload is occurring and that some preventative action should be taken. There is another even more important aspect of this behaviour. Since mechanical work is the force applied to the body multiplied by the distance (or deformation) that occurs under the influence of that load, it can be seen that the work (or energy) required to bring about fracture in a material is the area under a stress–strain (load–deformation) graph. Compare two materials (Fig. A.8) which have the same strength and the same Young's modulus. Ostensibly there may, on that basis, seem little to choose between them. However, the important point is that (A) is brittle and has no yield point, whereas (B) is ductile and because of its large range of plastic deformation before fracture has a much bigger area under its graph which indicates that it requires vastly more energy to cause catastrophic failure. Such a material has the toughness necessary for devices that may have to withstand impact loading.

BASIS FOR MATERIAL CHOICE

These factors illustrate the need to consider carefully all the physical parameters of a material before making a choice. In an ideal world manufacturers would publish stress/strain curves for all materials. Unfortunately, this does not happen and information is usually given in tabular form with ductility quoted as percentage elongation (i.e. the percentage increase in specimen length at the point of fracture). Thus the main factors governing material choice would be:

1. Ultimate strength (usually tensile).
2. Yield strength (usually tensile).
3. Young's modulus.
4. Percentage elongation.

It is interesting to compare some of the materials commonly used in orthotics. Stress–strain curves for steel and aluminium alloy are shown in Fig. A.9, from

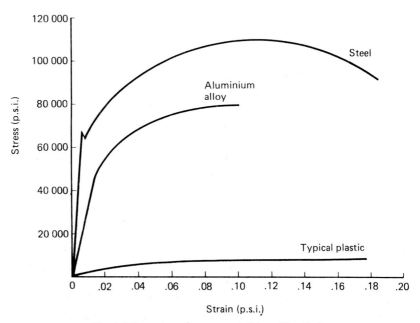

Fig. A.9 Comparison of common materials used in orthotics.

which it can be seen that steel is stronger and stiffer than aluminium alloy. However, it is well known that aluminium alloy has a much lower density (i.e. it is lighter) and for that reason is considered by many as preferable for lower limb orthotics, except when patients are described as heavy and/or vigorous.

If this choice was based purely on ultimate strength a larger aluminium alloy section could be used to produce a device that would compensate for lower strength of aluminium alloy and still be lighter than an equivalent steel orthosis. However, energy to failure is critically important for patients who predispose to orthotic failure and it is for this reason as much as strength that steel is specified for the highly active group. The comparison of area under the stress–strain curves shows how much more 'safe' steel is in this respect. When there is an additional requirement for high stiffness then steel has a further big advantage over aluminium alloy.

HEAT TREATMENT

The properties of metals can be altered by heat treatment. High-carbon steels can be made harder by cooling them rapidly from red heat in water. Whilst this can make them stronger, it also renders them very brittle and therefore unsuitable for orthotic applications. A compromise between the hard brittle condition and a soft ductile one can be achieved by different types of heat treatment in which temperature and rate of cooling are significant factors.

Clearly, care must be exercised during orthotic manufacturing processes to ensure that the carefully produced condition of such materials is not affected. Excessive heat will alter the properties of steels, and is also critical with aluminium alloys which are weakened at comparatively low temperatures. There is good reason for the DHSS ban on nylon-coated aluminium alloys; the material is weakened by the temperatures to which it is subjected during nylon dipping.

VISCO-ELASTIC BEHAVIOUR

A plastic material, polypropylene, has been shown on the same graph of stress–strain as the two metals discussed above (Fig. A.9). This shows that it is much more flexible (i.e. less stiff) and is considerably less strong. It has different advantages which will be discussed later. However, although it has been shown on a stress–strain graph for general comparison purposes, it is not entirely appropriate that this should be done. Plastics, in common with biological materials, exhibit visco-elastic behaviour which means that their physical properties vary depending on the rate at which the material is strained. This has implications for devices produced from these materials. When a visco-elastic material is strained to a particular level (say 2 per cent strain) and held at that level, then the stress produced within the material will gradually diminish with time (Fig. A.10). Although this may initially seem advantageous it must be remembered that the stress induced in the material is a measure of its resistance to applied force at the strain level considered. Thus what actually happens in visco-elastic materials is that their ability to resist force diminishes the longer a strain level is maintained. At the end of the day a plastic AFO is less effective than it was at the beginning.

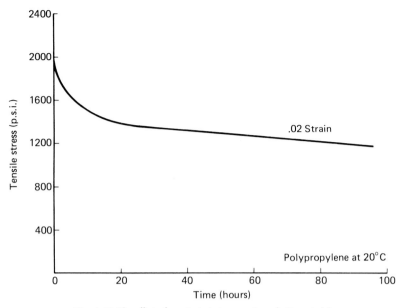

Fig. A.10 The effect of constant strain on a visco-elastic material.

One of the problems with visco-elastic materials is that it is very difficult to make comparisons of their physical properties. Published data are for specified strain rates and may not be relevant to the application under consideration because the strain rate may be different, or more likely, highly variable in nature. Detailed and comprehensive data on many plastics are published (Ogorkiewicz, 1970) but can be highly confusing except to a specialist in materials technology.

Another factor that causes significant variations in the performance of plastic materials is ambient temperature. The change in yield strength of polypropylene with temperature is shown in Fig. A.11 from which it will be seen that it can diminish by as much as 50 per cent in the range 0–40°C.

Despite these difficulties plastic materials play an extremely important role in the provision of orthotic care. They have advantages over metal in that they can be moulded to a cast of patient shape which provides a more closely fitting device that is quicker and easier to manufacture. With some plastics it is even possible to mould directly on the patient. Moulding to the patient shape is said, in many cases, to be more cosmetic in that there is little additional bulk. However, this also means that the structural properties are being governed by the patient rather than the designer, not always to the advantage of the patient.

FATIGUE

The definition of strength as stress at failure for a single cycle test is important because repeated loading causes materials to fail at a stress somewhat lower than their quoted strength. The effect of cyclic loading is to cause materials to

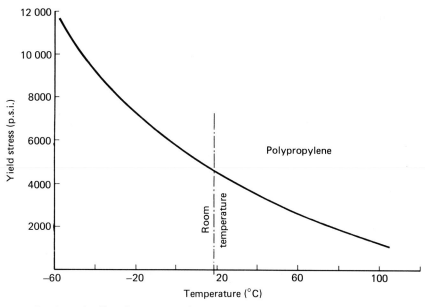

Fig. A.11 The effect of variation in ambient temperature on yield stress in polypropylene.

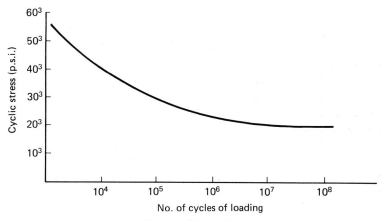

Fig. A.12 Fatigue failure.

weaken, and failure at the consequently lower stress level is known as fatigue failure. Several factors have a bearing on the number of cycles of loading necessary to cause fatigue failure. Clearly the higher the level of stress the lower the number of cycles to failure. Plotting stress against number of cycles (Fig. A.12) shows that this produces a curve which gradually 'flattens out' to the level of stress at which the material in question becomes virtually immune to fatigue failure. Where the stress changes from compressive to tensile in each cycle then a further reduction in fatigue life will occur.

Looked at in practical terms it is useful to realize that steel, for example, will withstand millions of cycles of loading when stress levels are kept to less than half the yield point. However, when stress levels are close to yield point the number of cycles to cause failure drops to thousands.

To put this into a useful context it is worth remembering that a normal person uses approximately 1 million gait cycles per annum. Clearly a lower limb orthosis should not be stressed above half the yield point of the material used in its structure if it is to last a reasonable length of time.

Fatigue is a problem for all classes of material. Some are more able to resist cyclic loading than others, but none is immune to fatigue failure. Steps can be taken to reduce the possibility of its occurrence during manufacture of a device. Poor surface finish in the form of scratches or notches, or sudden changes of section, all have the effect of producing a 'stress raiser' in the material (Fig. A.13). At such a point the stress level is much higher than the level of general stress in that section of the material. These higher stress levels cause fatigue failure to commence in the minute area at which the 'raiser' has an effect, and this causes the failure to spread gradually across the section. This is obviously an accelerating process because as it occurs it causes the 'general' stress level to rise as the material section becomes effectively smaller.

Thus it can be seen that whilst it is pleasing to have a nice surface finish on orthotic devices, it has a greater importance in reducing the risk of early structural failure due to fatigue. This cannot be over-emphasized. There is little point in hiding poor surface finish by coating the device with a finishing material such as paint. The stress raisers will still be there working away at diminishing the life of the orthosis, with potentially dangerous consequences for the patients. All classes of material require a good surface finish to minimize the risk of fatigue failure. Cut marks and notches in plastic orthoses should be smoothed out before they are supplied to patients.

STRUCTURES

Bending

One of the commonest forms of loading in orthotics is bending. This is particularly true with lower limb devices where the aim is to stabilize 'flail' joints. Ground-reaction forces produce moments about these joints and the orthosis provides the equal and opposite reacting moment which ensures that intrinsic stabilization is maintained. The stresses set up within the material of the orthosis are dependent not only on the area of the section (as with direct axial or

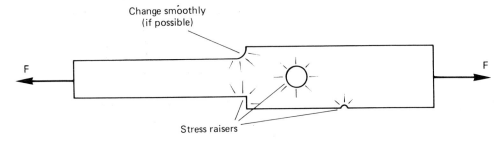

Fig. A.13 Typical stress raisers encountered in orthotics.

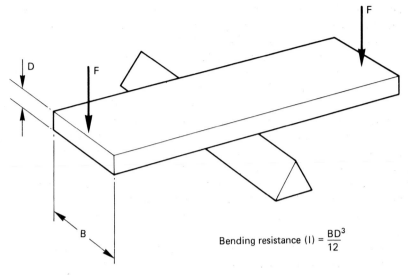

Bending resistance (I) $= \dfrac{BD^3}{12}$

Fig. A.14 Bending resistance (I) of flat plates.

shear loading) but also on the distribution of the material about the bending axis. This has important implications in the design, manufacture and clinical modification of orthoses. The resistance to bending of a rectangular section increases in proportion to its thickness cubed and directly with increases in its width (Fig. A.14). If a section is doubled in thickness, bending resistance is increased by a factor of eight, whereas doubling the width only doubles the bending resistance.

The importance of material distribution to bending resistance can be gauged by bending a flat plastic rule by hand about planes at 90 degrees. It is very easy to achieve large deflections about the flat plane, but almost impossible to bring about noticeable changes at 90 degrees to this. In both cases the area of material resisting the bending loads is exactly the same; the only difference is the distribution of material about the bending axis.

Material sections in bending

The shape of sections used in orthoses has a very significant bearing on their ability to withstand the bending loads which are so common, and the design of the structure must take account of the service requirements and the manufacturing techniques employed. Two commonly employed material sections for metal orthoses are half-round section and rectangular bevel-edge section (Fig. A.15(a) and (b)). Comparing the bending resistance of these two with a square section of the same area about the axis indicated shows that the figure for the half-round section is 12 per cent greater. On that basis alone the choice between them is easy. However, to produce an orthotic structure from these materials it is necessary for them to be joined to other components (e.g. knee joints) and material sections. This will necessitate the drilling of holes for

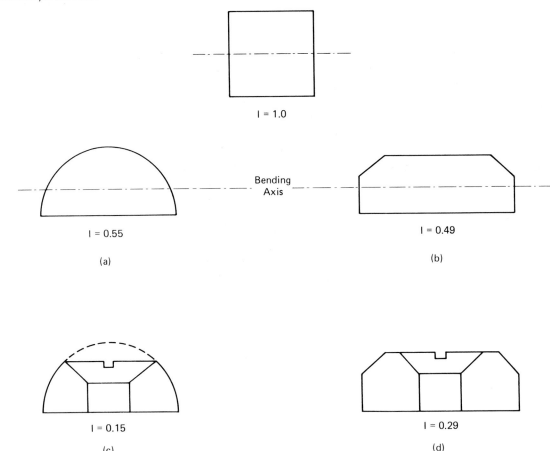

Fig. A.15 Comparison of the bending resistance (I) of common material sections used in orthotics.

screws or rivets and usually these require to be countersunk. When this is done the bending resistance of the section at the point where the hole is drilled will be affected, and the relationship of bending resistance to thickness cubed which previously seemed a great advantage can suddenly have a deleterious effect.

Comparing the half-round and rectangular bevel-edge sections with a countersunk hole drilled across the bending axis (Fig. A.15(c) and (d)) shows a dramatic change in their respective bending resistance. The half-round section now has only half that of the rectangular bevel-edge section because the countersink has removed material at the point where it is most effective in resisting bending. Since any device is only as strong as its weakest point, it can be seen that the method of manufacture is as important as selection of material and the shape of its section.

Moulded sections

Modern plastics which can mould to casts or directly on the patient use the shapes produced and the modification of these to achieve the desired structural properties. When flat material is moulded into a curved section the bending resistance is increased very significantly because the relationship in which small increases in thickness of the section bring about large increases in bending resistance works in favour of the structure (Fig. A.16).

A common plastic orthosis is a below-knee device moulded to a cast of the patient and modified to achieve particular structural requirements. In one embodiment the objective is to control plantar flexion of a mobile equinus deformity during swing phase, but to permit dorsi-flexion during stance phase in order to produce a natural gait pattern. This is achieved by moulding to a cast and cutting the trim lines to leave a section with just sufficient rigidity to control the equinus which then permits flexibility for dorsi-flexion. The material qualities necessary are provided by such materials as Ortholen, Sub-ortholen and polypropylene (the last two often requiring additional stiffening

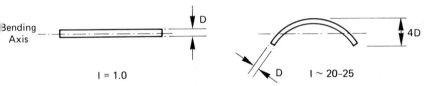

Fig. A.16 The effect on bending resistance (I) of moulding flat sections.

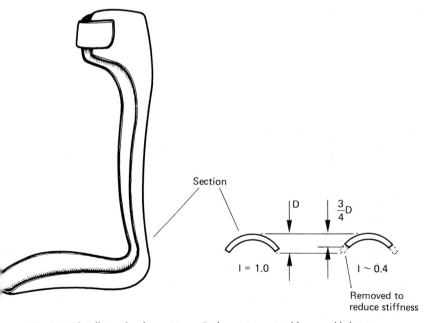

Fig. A.17 The effect on bending resistance (I) of removing material from moulded sections.

behind the Achilles tendon), all of which have good fatigue resistance and relatively good strength and stiffness.

The stiffness of this orthosis can be reduced by the orthotist at the fitting stage by trimming the narrow part of the orthosis, at which point it flexes. Care must be exercised in performing that adjustment because the laws of bending apply to the curved flat section of the material (Fig. A.17). Small amounts of material removed from the outer edges will reduce the effective bending section more than might initially be expected, and with bending resistance being related to the cube of bending-section thickness, the flexibility of the orthosis can be drastically reduced by careless removal of material.

A further application of the moulding technique might be to produce a fixed ankle, and in this case the moulding will need to be carried around the ankle, closer to the malleoli, in order to produce the additional stiffness to oppose dorsi-flexion during stance phase (Fig. A.18). This more complex shape will require the better moulding characteristics of polypropylene, even though the physical properties of Ortholen might be more suited to the application. Fatigue will again be a problem with the cyclic loading which will be encountered and this means that the even better moulding characteristics of polythene cannot be employed because this material has poor fatigue resistance.

Static applications such as wrist splints and some spinal jackets in which the complexity of moulding is an important consideration can utilize the advantages of polythene to good effect because fatigue is not a problem that will be encountered.

A disadvantage of producing orthoses by moulding to casts of the patient is that the shape of the structure is not always in the control of the designer. With a plastic AFO the shape of the shank has a significant bearing on the performance of the device. This design has been developed to provide acceptable

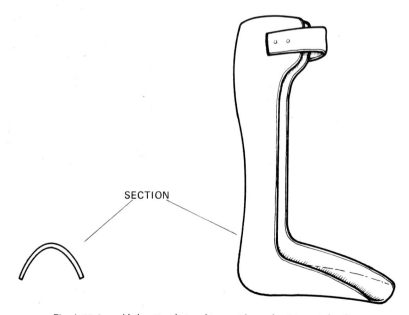

SECTION

Fig. A.18 A moulded section designed to provide good resistance to bending.

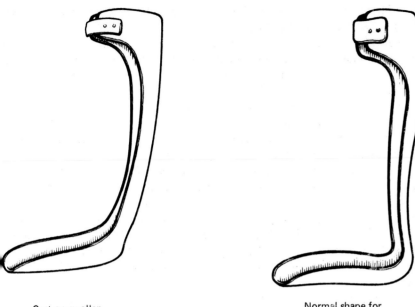

Cast on swollen
shank

Normal shape for
the orthosis

Fig. A.19 The possible effect of patient shape on orthotic performance in moulded sections.

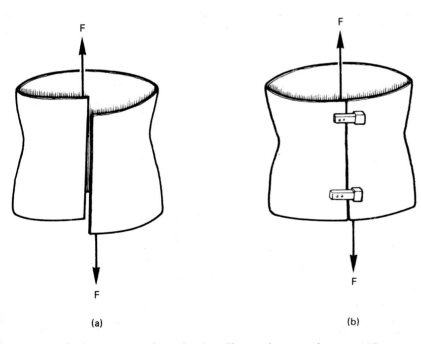

(a)

(b)

Fig. A.20 The improvement that can be achieved by providing stuctural integrity. (a) Poor resistance to deformation. (b) Improved resistance by bracing across the split to give some structural integrity.

performance with a normally shaped shank, but some patients may have a deformity that adversely affects the structural properties that are obtained. An example of this is shown in an AFO produced from a cast of a polio victim with gross swelling at the back of the ankle (Fig. A.19) (see page 147).

Structural integrity

The most rigid type of structure is one that is completely integral. A tube is a common example and demonstrates the advantage of such structures. Not only does it resist bending along its length, it also resists torsion about its axis. This integrity of structure can be important in orthotics but is difficult to achieve if patients are to be able to doff and don their apparatus. Some spinal orthoses require the overall structural properties of a tube, but of necessity must be split for the patient to gain access. The split in the 'tube' diminishes its ability to stabilize the spine because integrity is lost and it becomes easy to deform the structure (the edges of the split can be moved relative one to another along their length with comparative ease) (Fig. A.20(a)). Some of the structural integrity can be regained by securing the orthosis on the patient with locating devices which are themselves rigid and therefore able to prevent the edges of the orthosis moving relative to each other (Fig. A.20(b)) (see Fig. 5.7, page 44).

Material selection

There is clearly a relationship between the materials selected and the type of structures used for given requirements. Many factors must be balanced if a satisfactory compromise is to be achieved. This is true of all structural design exercises, but is complicated in orthotics by the additional factors encountered by having to fit devices to patients. Cosmesis is considered important, but the physical interreactions of pressure and adverse skin reaction can have overriding implications. It is helpful to bear in mind the advantages of the two main groups of materials used for structural purposes in orthotics:

1. Plastics:
    (a) Light weight.
    (b) Mouldability.
    (c) Resistance to chemical attack.
    (d) Ease of fabrication and moulding.
    (e) Cosmetic (?).
2. Metals:
    (a) High strength.
    (b) High stiffness.
    (c) Stable characteristics at ambient temperatures.
    (d) High-energy absorption before failure.

For many applications the choice of materials will be obvious. In other situations there will be no absolutely correct choice and the advantage of the two groups must be balanced against the requirements of the application.

FAIL–SAFE DESIGN

Even when great care is exercised in selecting appropriate materials, designing orthoses for the function intended and finishing components to minimize the possibility of fatigue failure, it must be recognized that because of the varied activities of patients, overload of devices is always a possibility. Dynamic loading of orthotic devices by patients who are very active can mean much higher stress levels. Even slow ambulation, for example, can produce forces in the lower limbs which are 20–30 per cent higher than body weight. Vigorous swing-through gait could increase the forces to 2–3 times body weight and jumping off kerbs and steps to 5–8 times body weight. All of these additional forces will bring about commensurate increases in stress levels in the orthoses worn by such patients. Since their safety is of paramount importance orthoses should incorporate fail–safe features as far as it is possible to do so because the dynamic forces of unforeseen activity can lead to severe overloading. Clearly, selection of materials will play a part in this and those that are ductile and have high energy absorption before fracture are to be much preferred. Additionally 'back up' devices should be employed and it is for this reason as much as function that stops are fitted to both joints in calipers with double side members.

ORTHOTIC DESIGN FACTORS

Material properties and structural design are inextricably interrelated. Proper account of the effects of one on the other is essential if poor design and practice in orthotics is to be avoided. An important aspect of manufacture is the verification of material specification. Alterations in material content can have important implications which the producer might not appreciate. Polypropylene in its pure state has excellent properties for plastic orthoses. However, it is sometimes 'diluted' with other materials and this causes early failure.

Manufacturing processes must also be carefully controlled. Heat treatment on metals has been discussed, but it must also be remembered that overheating plastics during moulding can seriously affect their mechanical properties and cause the device being produced to be of unacceptable quality.

All aspects of material selection, structural design, manufacturing processes, quality of finish and care of the finished device will affect the suitability and durability of orthotic devices. They must all be carefully considered if successful treatment is to be provided for patients who require orthotic assistance.

RECOMMENDED READING

Campbell, G., Newell, E. and McLure, M. (1982). Compression testing of foamed plastics and rubbers for use as orthotic shoe insoles. *Prosth. Orth. Int.* **6**, 48–52.

Condie, D. N. and Meadows, C. B. (1977). Some biomechanical considerations in the design of ankle–foot orthoses. *Orthot. Prosthet.* **31**, 45–52.

Dumbleton, H. H. and Black, J. (1975). *An Introduction to Orthopaedic Materials.* Springfield, Il.: Charles C. Thomas.

Gordon, J. E. (1968). *The New Science of Strong Materials or Why Things Do Not Fall Through the Floor.* Harmondsworth: Penguin Original.

Gordon, J. E. (1978). *Structures or Why Things Don't Fall Down.* Harmondsworth: Penguin Original.

Lautenschlager, E. P., Bayne, S. C., Wildes, R., Russ, J. C. and Yanke, M. J. (1975). Materials investigation of failed plastic orthoses. *Orthot. Prosthet.* **29**, 25–7.

Lipskin, R. (1971). Materials in orthotics. *Bull. Prosthet. Res.* **Spring**, 107–22.

Nicholas, J. J., Carven, H., Weiner, G., Crawshaw, C. and Taylor, F. (1982). Splinting in rheumatoid arthritis: evaluation of Lightcast II fibreglass polymer splints. *Arch. Phys. Med. Rehab.* **63**, 95.

Ogorkiewicz, R. M. (Ed.). (1970). *Engineering Properties of Thermoplastics.* New York: Wiley-Interscience.

Robin, G. C., Magora, A., Adler, E. and Saltiel, J. (1968). Dynamic stress analysis of below-knee drop foot braces. *Med. Biol. Eng.* **6**, 533–46.

Rubin, G. and Dixon, M. (1973). The modern ankle–foot orthoses (AFOs). *Bull. Prosthet. Res.* **Spring**, 20–41.

Shimeld, A., Campbell, G. and Ernest, M. (1982). An interdisciplinary methodology for the comparative evaluation of splinting materials. *Can. J. Occupat. Ther.* **49**, 79–83.

Appendix B: Biomechanics of the foot

Traditionally the starting point for the consideration of the functional anatomy of the foot has been to compare it with a static structure such as a bridge.
This approach detracts from understanding more than it reveals and makes no
allowance for the fact that in usage, the foot is a highly mobile structure in all
planes, with a wide range of adaptability to allow for variations in ground
shape and slope.

In one respect, there is an analogy between a bridge and the foot, namely
that both are made up of multiple segments which are held together by appropriate structures to resist the mechanical stresses of the full range of function.
To understand the similarities and differences it is essential to have a clear
understanding of the term arch and beam.

An arch is a structure, the ends of which when loaded tend to move apart
and are prevented from doing so either by stops placed at each end (Fig.
B.1(a)), which is clearly not the case in a foot, or by a tie placed between the
ends (Fig. B.1(b)). If, as is correct, the load-bearing structure of the foot when
standing must be regarded as from the metatarsal heads to the os calcis there is
no strictly comparable structure to such a tie. The plantar aponeurosis (see Fig.
3.19, page 33) does arise at one end, the os calcis, but passes beyond the
metatarsal end to be attached into the proximal phalanges. If the toes are prevented from flexing by apposition with the floor it can then act as a tie (Fig.
B.1(c)). The ease with which the toes can be raised from the floor actively
when in this position indicates that the tension in the aponeurosis is low and
its effect as a tie is slight.

A beam, which can be either a single structure or segmented, resists deformation by the strength of the material of which it is constructed. In the foot
this is the bone and the strong and strategically placed ligaments beneath the
bone, which are tense at the time of application of load. There is within this
structure a combination of tension and compression (Fig. B.2).

Whilst it is completely established that no muscle action is required to maintain the posture of the normal foot, the muscles, working intermittently, serve
to relieve the stress on these structures and help in the absorption of shock. In
the abnormal they may be called upon to work more or less continuously. This
can be a cause of pain, fatigue or even tendon rupture.

If the foot rolls inwards, as in pronation, the relationship of these strong
stress-supporting ligaments and muscles to the joints and to the line of action
of the stress is altered adversely and in gross pronation the spring ligament

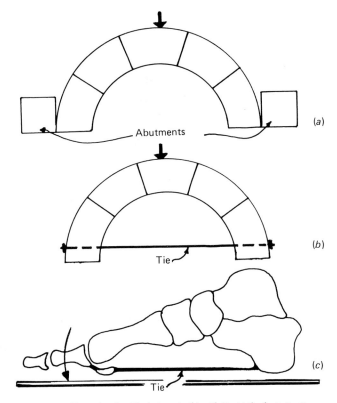

Fig. B.1 (a) Typical arch with abutments; (b) with tie; (c) the foot situation.

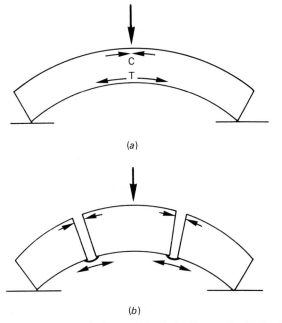

Fig. B.2 (a) Curved beam. (b) Segmented beam. C = Compression; T = tension.

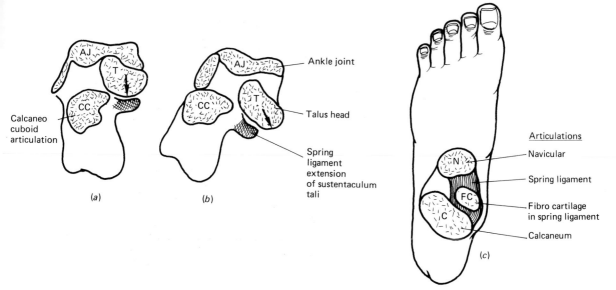

Fig. B.3 Transverse section of the foot through the mid-tarsal joint. (a) Normal posture showing position of sustentaculum tali with extension forward of the spring ligament in the normal position, supporting the head of the talus. (b) Pronated, showing the inefficient support of the talar head which is pushing downwards and rotating inwards against the weak medial capsule. (c) View from above of spring ligament.

(plantar calcaneo-navicular), passing as it does from the front of the os calcis to the under-surface of the navicular bone and supporting the head of the talus, rotates laterally. The stresses will then come more on the medial capsule of the talonavicular joint, which is not designed to sustain these and which will in consequence give rise to pain and/or stretch (Fig. B.3).

ARTICULATIONS

The dynamic mobility of the foot derives from the nature of the articulations, a word which includes joints but is not limited to these.

They are of two types: intrinsic and extrinsic.

Intrinsic

These are hinge-type cartilage covering low-friction joints rotating about a single axis and are, therefore, track bound. Like a door on its hinge they can rotate only clockwise or anticlockwise about the axis of the joint, in this case the centre pin of the hinge (Fig. B.4(a)). Anatomically the axis is the product of

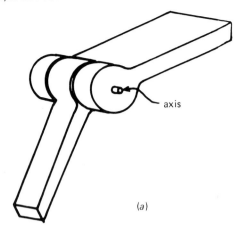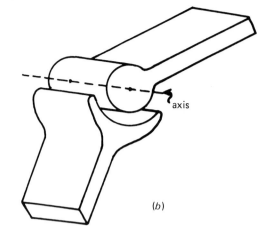

(a)   (b)

Fig. B.4 Hinge articulations.

the joint shape held in contact by ligaments (Fig. B.4(b)). All joints of the foot, including the ankle, are of this type and together form a track-bound linkage which moves with a set pattern no matter at what point or in what direction force is applied, e.g. external rotation of the leg produces a supination of the foot with the ankle moving laterally; and internal rotation, the opposite effect of pronation with changes in the weight-bearing area of the foot (Fig. B.5). In the normal foot because of the shape and distribution of ligaments of the major joints concerned, particularly the subtalar, pronation is small in range and supination considerable. However, in the abnormal foot, e.g. the hyper-mobile foot (see page 125), where the range is increased, problems of instability will occur as shown later.

The position of these axes in space is important. That of the subtalar axis (Fig. B.6) transmits the side-to-side movement of the foot to rotational movements of the leg and simultaneously there will be a distal rotation of the meta-tarso-phalangeal joint of the great toe relative to the ground. Where this is considerable there will be an adverse ground reaction tending to push the toe into the valgus position (Fig. B.7) and this accounts for the higher incidence of hallux valgus which occurs with abnormally pronated feet.

Extrinsic

These are not joints but are high-friction rolling articulations beneath the under-surface of the os calcis and the metatarsal heads within the immensely valuable specialized fibro-fatty tissue between these and the skin.

The axis in Fig. B.8 moves in space, like that of a bicycle wheel over the ground, relative to the skin, which is stationary, and in this respect there is an analogy between the wheels of an army tank which move in space whilst the track remains stationary in relationship to the ground contact. The shear-absorbing function of this arrangement has been noted (see Fig. 2.6, page 15). This articulation is not track bound and can move in any plane.

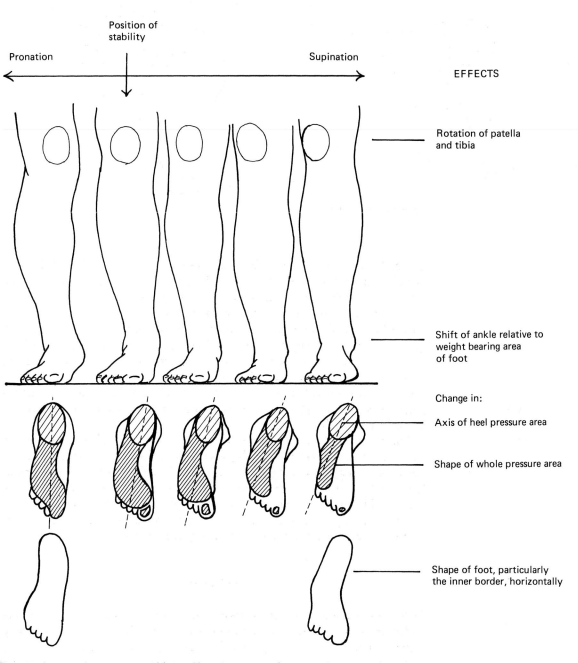

Fig. B.5 Changes to be seen in a normal foot and leg on pronation and supination.

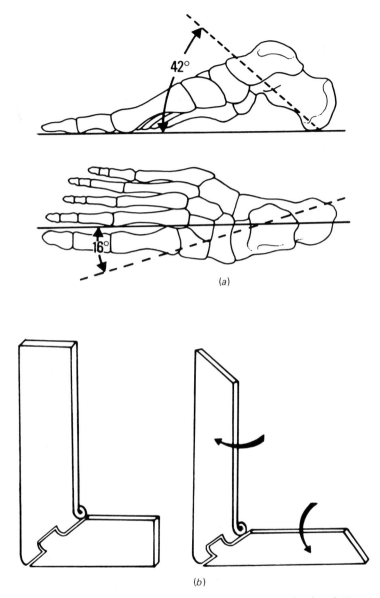

Fig. B.6 (a) Average position of the subtalar axis in space to the standing foot. (b) Torque transmission effect of rotation from leg to foot and vice versa.

If the foot is moved from side to side when held in the air the simple hinge action of the intrinsic joints can be observed, but if the foot is now placed on the ground and rolled inwards and outwards movement becomes much more complex as there is now a compound action of the intrinsic and extrinsic articulations.

Beneath the subtalar joint the foot can be compared to a six-legged stool, five legs anteriorly (the metatarsal rays), and one posteriorly (the os calcis). It is a specialized stool in that the anterior rays are articulated both at the navicular-

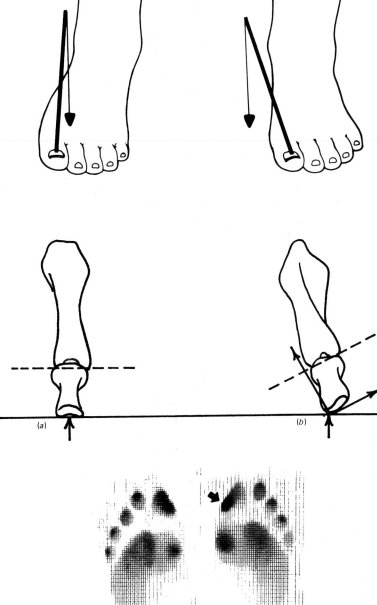

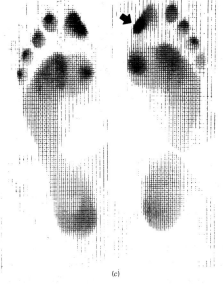

Fig. B.7 Change in spatial position of the metatarso-phalangeal joint of the great toe and effect of the ground reaction from (a) normal to (b) pronated foot with valgus producing deformity from the great toe. This is reflected in rotation of great toe nail which is also seen in differential footprint (c).

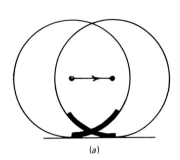

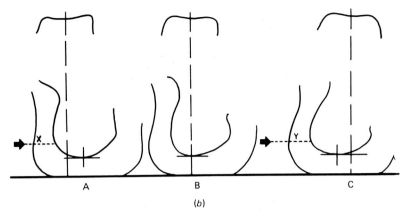

Fig. B.8 Lateral rolling articulation of os calcis. (a) Diagrammatic. (b) Movement seen on radiograph from the fixed arrow: A is pronation; B is normal standing posture; and C is supination.

cuneiform joints and at those at the bases of the metatarsals. This structure is inherently stable when loaded and these joints are then in full extension. This is in fact a unique situation in the body as at no other place are the joints expected to function continuously at the extreme range with a continuous mechanical stress on the supporting ligaments. Clearly, hypermobility, either inherent or due to disease in these joints, can affect the posture of the foot.

For visualization it is easier to consider the foot as a three-legged stool (Fig. B.9). The ideal stable state is that the load should be applied to fall within the support area so that the forces in each stool leg are equal, and clinically this can be designated a balanced stable foot. However, if, as in Fig. B.10, the load moves away from this position but still remains within the support area, an unbalanced stable foot will occur (Rose, 1982). This will mean that there is a mal-distribution of weight in the support area, a potential extrinsic pressure stress problem. A beneficial effect of the lateral rolling of the os calcis on pronation and supination is that it moves the posterior joint of the support area, and tends, therefore, to keep the load line within this area (Fig. B.11).

Should the load move further to one side, the line of application will pass outside the support area and in the case of the stool it will tip over to lie on its side in another stable position. This is called metastability in engineering terms and such a foot can be described as metastable (Fig. B.12) and will produce intrinsic stress problems.

In the foot, of course, the top of the stool is linked through the subtalar joint to the tibia and what then happens very much depends on the range of available mobility in a particular foot. In the normal foot, as indicated, pronation is very limited and metastability does not occur but in the hypermobile foot there may be a situation in which the end of the range of movement in the subtalar joint is reached and is the limiting factor. In such circumstances abnormal stresses are placed on the ligaments and capsule on the inner side, with resultant symptoms. The wider range of supination of the foot means that the metastable position can be reached normally. This puts great stresses on the lateral ligaments of the ankle joint and will commonly, when these are high

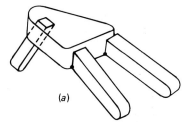

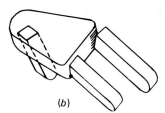

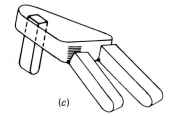

Fig. B.9 The subtalar stool, here represented for clarity with only two anterior legs, the first and fifth metatarsals. (a) The articulations at the bases of the metatarsal rays are fully extended and the stool stable. (b) and (c) When pronated or supinated the articulation towards which the movement is made remains closed whilst the others open differentially. Provided the load line remains within the support area, when the forces producing these movements are removed the stool will return to the normal resting position with all joints closed.

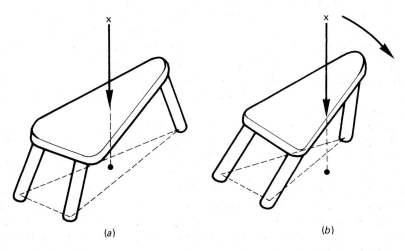

Fig. B.10 Load line (X) in relationship to support area. (a) The stool is stable. In (b) the stool rotates on to its side; a metastable position.

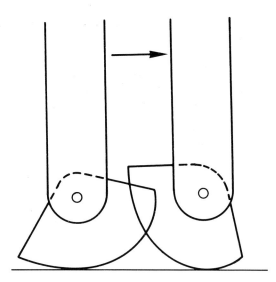

Fig. B.11 Diagram to illustrate the movement of the contact area at the os calcis articulation which tends to keep the load line within the support area.

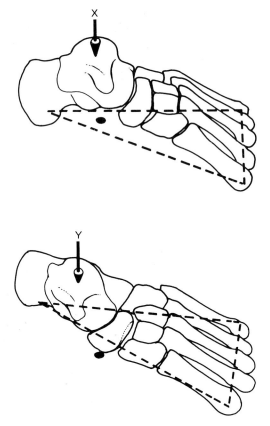

Fig. B.12 Load line (X) falls within the support area; Load line (Y) is outside the support area and produces a metastable foot. Note coincident change in the shape of the foot.

and sudden, cause tearing of these, accompanied by fractures, initially of the external malleolus and subsequently of the posterior tibial articulation (Rose, 1963).

If made up into a model as represented in Fig. B.13, the characteristics of the foot when standing can be demonstrated. The model can be used to identify certain important orthotic concepts, which can then be tested clinically:

1. The inherent stability of a normal foot.
2. That correction of the shoe-covered foot can be monitored by the rotation of the tibia.
3. That using this method it can be demonstrated that a wedge placed medially under the shoe heel causes no correction (Rose, 1958, 1962) (Fig. B.14). Of course, doing this does rotate the inner side of the upper of the shoe to press in a corrective fashion against the foot, but as is well shown clinically it is the upper that distorts and not the foot that corrects. A raise under the inner border of the sole and the heel does produce beneficial results for as long as this raise remains unworn.
4. That a corrective force for a pronated foot needs to be applied as a moment arm about the subtalar axis which itself had moved in space with the deformation of the foot (Fig. B.15).
5. That a metastable type of foot, brought into the corrected position, becomes stable and requires no significant interface retaining force.
6. That if the first metatarsal is shortened this will cause pronation of the foot, where the subtalar range allows this. It may not affect the function of the foot. About 30 per cent of the population show reduced support under the first metatarsal head (Fig. B.16) with no apparent ill effect. There is increased load under the pulp of the great toe, and this requires greater than normal activity of the long flexor muscle. Only if the narrowed forefoot support produces an unbalanced stable or metastable foot will there be a disability.

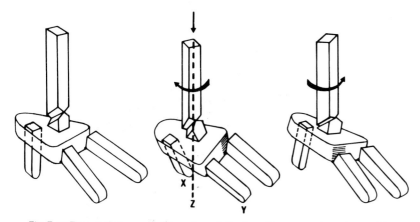

Fig. B.13 Diagrammatic representation of a model to show the compound interaction of the subtalar stool and the subtalar articulation.

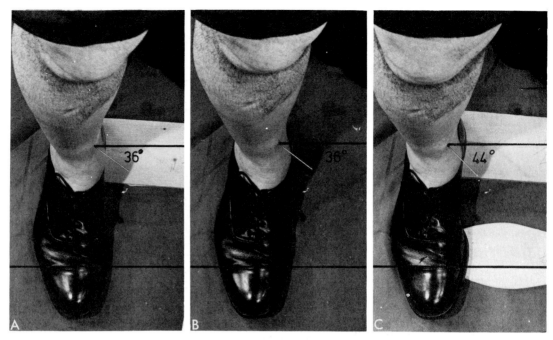

Fig. B.14 A metal pin driven into the tibia (B) shows the angle between this and a standard baseline in an unaltered shoe. (A) shows that there is no tibial rotation with a 6.35 mm (¼ in) raise under the heel only, whereas in (C) a raise under the inner sole and heel produces supination of the foot and rotation of the tibia.

Fig. B.15 Arrows indicate the point of application and direction of the most efficient corrective force to stabilize the corrected foot in the normal (N) position, and to initiate stabilization of the pronated foot (P). Hence the use of an inside Y-strap and outside iron (see Fig. 13.4, page 129). The distally extended heel cup acts similarly (see Fig. 13.6, page 131).

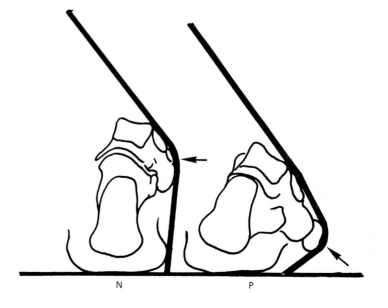

N   P

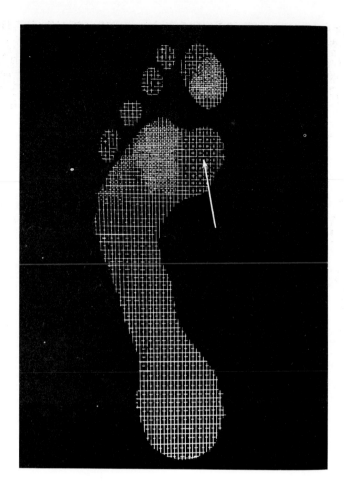

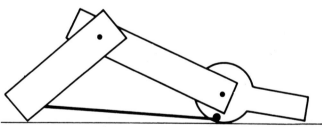

Fig. B.16 A differential pressure footmat shows reduced support under the first metatarsal head (arrow). In this case there was increased pressure under the second metatarsal and under the pulp of the great toe.

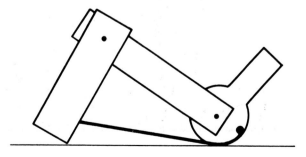

Fig. B.17 The 'windlass' effect of tightening the slip of plantar aponeurosis by extending a proximal phalanx, causing arch rise.

PLANTAR APONEUROSIS

This is a very important structure functionally (see Fig. 3.19, page 33). Extension of the phalanx to which each slip is attached has a 'windlass' effect (Fig. B.17).

This causes the longitudinal arch of that ray slip to rise, maximally in the first ray and negligibly in the fifth. This in turn supinates the foot and then through the track-bound linkage causes the effects already noted, namely external rotation of the tibia. The shock-absorbing mechanism on heel-strike and the foot-stabilizing effect on heel raise to toe-off has already been discussed, but importantly it has now been established that the great toe extension test is the most useful single sign in demonstrating an abnormal foot (Rose and Welton, 1985). With the patient standing erect and looking forward, the feet slightly apart, the examiner pushes the great toe into extension; in the normal foot, arch rise and tibial rotation will occur. With the slightly abnormal foot, arch rise only will occur; and with the profoundly abnormal foot neither is demonstrated.

This is a most important concept; namely, that abnormality of the foot should be judged by functional testing and not by inspection and description.

In order to investigate this viewpoint, the Valgus index was measured on 177 children between the ages of 5 and 7, the entire contents of two infant schools, and this investigation was recently repeated with essentially similar results.

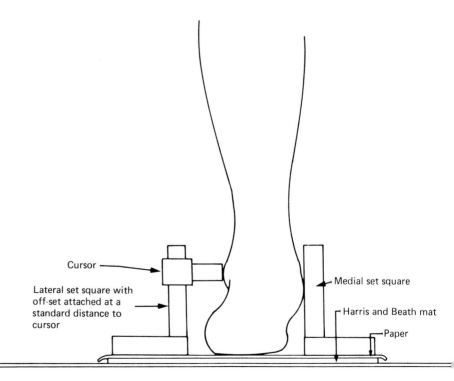

Fig. B.18 Method of measuring Valgus index.

The Valgus index is measured by projecting downwards from the standing foot the intermalleolar diameter on to a differential pressure mat (Harris and Beath, 1947) which records the footprint (Fig. B.18). This measures the shift of the intermalleolar diameter in relation to the heel area, and by a simple formula this is corrected so that no matter what size the foot, the index is applicable (Fig. B.19). The results are shown in Fig. B.20. They demonstrate that the average index was 11, and it will be noted that there is a high index both in the low-arched and in the high-arched feet.

It was the conclusion of further research (Rose and Welton, 1985) that only where the index was over 20 and combined with an abnormal great toe extension test was the foot likely to be abnormal, no matter what the shape; and that the old criterion on abnormality, the so-called valgus heel, which was generally associated with a high index, was no longer tenable. The importance clinically is that the abnormal foot should be detected early and treated efficiently whilst the vastly greater proportion of functionally normal feet which 'looked abnormal', often treated inefficiently, should be eliminated from the clinic.

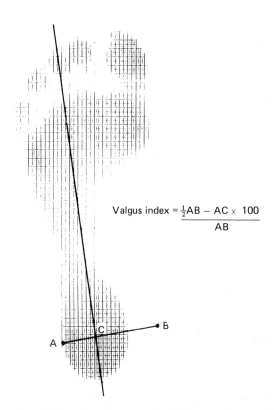

$$\text{Valgus index} = \frac{\frac{1}{2}AB - AC}{AB} \times 100$$

Fig. B.19 Calculation of Valgus index. AB = intermalleolar diameter; C = centre of heel contact area with line drawn through the middle toe.

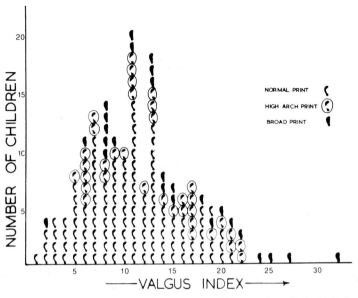

Fig. B.20 Distribution of the Valgus index (V.I.) in 177 children aged 5–7. Both with high-arch and with broad prints the index can be very high.

REFERENCES AND RECOMMENDED READING

Harris, R. J. and Beath, T. (1947). *Army Foot Survey—An Investigation of Foot Ailments in Canadian Soldiers.* Ottawa: National Research Council of Canada.

Hicks, J. H. (1951). The function of the plantar aponeurosis. *J. Anat.* **85**, 414.

Hicks, J. H. (1953). The mechanics of the foot. I. The joints. *J. Anat.* **87**, 354.

Hicks, J. H. (1954). The mechanics of the foot. II. The plantar aponeurosis and the arch. *J. Anat.* **88**, 25.

Hicks, J. H. (1955). The foot as a support. *Acta Anat.* **25**, 34.

Rose, G. K. (1958). Correction of the pronated foot. *J. Bone. Jnt. Surg.* **40B**, 674.

Rose, G. K. (1962). Correction of the pronated foot. *J. Bone. Jnt. Surg.* **44B**, 642.

Rose, G. K. (1963). Ankle injuries. In *Modern Trends in Orthopaedics*, Ed. J. M. P. Clark, p. 155. London: Butterworths.

Rose, G. K. (1982). Pes planus. In *Disorders of the Foot*, Ed. M. H. Jahss, p. 486. Philadelphia: W. B. Saunders.

Rose, G. K. and Welton, E. A. (1985). The diagnosis of flat foot in the child. *J. Bone Jnt. Surg.* **67B**, 172.

Index